I0135120

Improve Eyesight

Natural Ways to Improve Your Vision Fast

(Scientifically Proven Ways to Improve Your Eyesight Naturally)

Camille Wright

Published By **Simon Dough**

Camille Wright

All Rights Reserved

Improve Eyesight: Natural Ways to Improve Your Vision Fast (Scientifically Proven Ways to Improve Your Eyesight Naturally)

ISBN   978-1-77485-971-1

No part of this guidebook shall be reproduced in any form without permission in writing from the publisher except in the case of brief quotations embodied in critical articles or reviews.

Legal & Disclaimer

The information contained in this ebook is not designed to replace or take the place of any form of medicine or professional medical advice. The information in this ebook has been provided for educational & entertainment purposes only.

The information contained in this book has been compiled from sources deemed reliable, and it is accurate to the best of the Author's knowledge; however, the Author cannot guarantee its accuracy and validity and cannot be held liable for any errors or omissions. Changes are periodically made to this book. You must consult your doctor or get professional medical advice before using any of the suggested remedies, techniques, or information in this book.

Upon using the information contained in this book, you agree to hold harmless the Author from and against any damages, costs, and expenses, including any legal fees potentially resulting from the application of any of the information provided by this guide. This disclaimer applies to any damages or injury caused by the use and application, whether directly or indirectly, of any advice or information presented, whether for breach of contract, tort, negligence, personal injury, criminal intent, or under any other cause of action.

You agree to accept all risks of using the information presented inside this book. You need to consult a professional medical practitioner in order to ensure you are both able and healthy enough to participate in this program.

Table Of Contents

Chapter 1: Eye Problems

Many people have eye problems at one time or another. Some are minor and can be treated easily at home. Others will require specialist care.

There are many things you can do for your eyesight to improve, no matter how bad it is.

You might be experiencing any of these issues? Always consult your doctor if you experience severe symptoms or persist for more than a few weeks.

Eye strain

This condition is known to everyone who works long hours on a computer or reads for hours. It happens when you abuse your eyes. They can become tired and need rest as with any other body part.

If your eyes feel tired, take some time to relax. You should consult your doctor if you feel that your eyes are still feeling tired after a few weeks.

Your eyes appear so bloodshot. Why?

Your eyes' surface is covered with blood vessels, which grow when they're injured or inflamed. It gives your eyes a crimson look.

Eye strain may be a reason. Your doctor should be consulted if you suspect that there may have been an injury.

Red eyes can be a sign that you have another eye condition, such as conjunctivitis (pinkeye), sun damage or a lack of sunglasses. If the symptoms don't go away with rest and over-the counter eye drops, you should consult your doctor.

Night Blindness

Can you see well at night, especially when driving in dark? Is it difficult for you to navigate dark areas, such as movie theatres,?

That sounds like night blindness. It's only a symptom. Night blindness is caused by nearsightedness or cataracts, keratoconus or a lack thereof. These are all conditions that doctors may treat.

This condition may be inherited, or could develop from a degenerative retinal disease. Low light conditions will make it more difficult for those with the condition.

Lazy Eye

If one eye isn't growing normally, the lazy eye (or amblyopia) develops. This eye has poorer vision, and tends to move more slowly than the other. It is seen in infants, children, and the elderly. Rarely does it affect both eyes. It is essential to get treatment as soon as possible for children and newborns.

It is possible to avoid vision problems for the rest of your life if you catch a lazy-eye early in your child's life. Contact lenses or corrective glasses are available. The patch may also be used.

Cross Eyes (Strabismus), Nystagmus

If you notice that your eyes don't align properly when you look at anything, it could be strabismus. It might also be called "crossed eyes" or "walleye".

This problem is not going away on its' own. In some cases, an eye doctor may recommend vision therapy to help strengthen the weak eye muscles. It is common to need to see an ophthalmologist or expert in eye surgery to correct it. It will require a visit to an eye doctor or ophthalmologist to fix it.

Nystagmus means that the eye is constantly moving or "jiggles", and it can be triggered by a stimulus.

Vision therapy is a treatment that strengthens your eyes. Surgery is also an option. Your doctor will evaluate your eyes to determine which therapy is most effective for you.

Colorblindness

If you cannot see or differentiate between certain hues (usually reds and yellows), then you might be colorblind. This occurs when the color cells within your eyes (the doctor will refer to them as cone cells) become dysfunctional or missing.

You can only see in grays when the condition is severe. However, this is very rare. It affects about half of all people. You might get it later on in life if you take certain medicines or have other health conditions. Your doctor can help you determine the source. This condition is more common in males than in females.

An easy test will help you identify your condition. You can't get treatment if it's something you were born with, but special contacts and glasses are available to help people see the differences between hues.

Uveitis

This is the name for a group that causes inflammation of the uvea. It's the layer at the center of the eye that contains most of the blood vessels.

These disorders could cause vision loss or damage to eye tissue. You may experience it in people of different ages. It may be temporary or persistent.

Uveitis can be more common among people who have an immune system disorder such as AIDS or rheumatoid. These symptoms may include:

Blurred vision

Eye pain

Eye redness

Sensitivity towards light

If you are experiencing these symptoms, and they persist beyond a few days or longer, contact your doctor. There are many treatment options available for uveitis. The type of the disease you have will determine which one.

Presbyopia

This happens when you lose the ability, despite strong distant sight, to detect small objects and text.

For some people, reading a book or other type of material may be more difficult after the age of 40. Similar to your arms being too short.

You can restore your reading vision with contact lenses, reading glasses, or laser eye surgery LASIK.

Floaters

These are tiny dots or particles that appear to float around your field of view. They can be seen most often in brightly lit areas or outside on sunny days.

Floaters are typically benign, but they can be an indicator of more severe eye disease like retinal detachment. The retina at the back is what causes the layer below to separate from your eyes. As a result, light flashes can also occur along with floaters and black shadows appearing at the edges of your sight.

If you notice a sudden increase in the amount or frequency of spots, flashes, or a new "curtain", you should consult your eye doctor right away.

Dry Eyes

When your eyes stop producing enough quality tears, this is called a dry eye. This can cause you to feel that something is in your eyes or that it's burning. Only rarely, and in extreme cases, can excessive dryness cause loss of sight. Here are some options:

Use a humidifier inside your house

Special eye drops work just like real tears

You can plug your tear ducts with a plug to reduce drainage

Lipiflow is a treatment which uses heat and compression to treat dry eyes

Testosterone eyelid cream

Supplements with fish oil or omega-3

Dry eye disease can be diagnosed if you have persistent dry eyes. To stimulate tear production, your doctor may prescribe medicated drops such cyclosporine or Restasis (Cequa and Restasis) to help promote tear growth.

Excessive tearing

It has nothing to with your emotions. You may be sensitive or hypersensitive to light, wind, temperature changes, or both. Wear sunglasses to protect your eyes.

Tearing could also be an indication of a more serious condition, such as an infection or blocked tear duct. These disorders can be treated by your eye doctor.

Cataracts

These are hazy patches that develop in the eye lens.

A healthy lens has a clear, sharp image. Light passes through it to your retina. This is the part of your eye where photos are processed. Because of cataracts, light isn't able to pass as quickly. The result is that you may not be able to see well, and might experience glare around lights at night.

Cataracts develop usually slowly. They don't cause symptoms such as redness, discomfort, or tears.

Some are minor and do not affect your sight. Surgery can often help to correct any damage that may occur.

Glaucoma

Your eye is a tire. A little pressure inside it is natural and healthy. High levels can damage your visual nerve. Glaucoma can be described as a combination of several illnesses that causes this condition.

Primary open angle vision is the most common. Most people with it do not experience symptoms or discomfort. It's important to continue with your routine eye examinations.

Although it is not common, glaucoma can be caused by the following:

Eye injury

Blocked blood vessels

Treatment for inflammatory diseases of eyes includes prescription eye drops or surgery.

Retinal Disorders

The retina is a thin, transparent line at the back and center of your eye. It is made of cells that capture images and transmit them to your brain. Retinal disease can cause damage to the retinal cell and block this transmission. There are several types.

Age-related Macular Degeneration refers a loss of vision in the macula, a tiny area of the retina.

Diabetic retinopathy refers to damage of blood vessels in your retina due to diabetes.

When the retina separates from the layer below it, there is a condition called retina detachment.

It is vital to be treated promptly and receive a diagnosis.

Conjunctivitis, also known as Pinkeye. This condition is caused by inflammation of tissue that lines your eyelids behind your sclera. It could cause redness or itching, burning, irritation, discharge, or the sensation that something is inside your eye.

It can affect people of different ages. These can include allergic reactions, illness, and exposure to chemicals.

Regular hand washing will reduce your chance of getting it.

Corneal Diseases

The cornea is the transparent dome-shaped "window", located at the front and center of your eye. It helps to focus light entering the eye. It could be hurt by infection, injury, or being exposed to toxins. Here are some signs to look out for:

Red eyes

Watery eyes

Pain

Reduced eyesight or a "halo effect"

The main therapies include:

New prescription for contacts or eyeglasses

Medicated Eye Drops

Problems with the eyelids

Your eyelids do a lot for you. They protect your eye, help to disseminate tear fluid throughout the surface and reduce light entering.

Eyelid problems are often characterized by pain, itching and weeping. There may also be blinking spasms near your eyelashes.

It could involve medication, surgery, or adequate cleaning.

Vision Changes

As you get older you may notice that you don't have the same vision as before. That's normal. Contacts and glasses are likely. You might choose to have surgery (LASIK), to correct your eyesight. A stronger prescription might be necessary if you already have glasses.

Age can also lead to other serious health problems. Macular degeneration, glaucoma and cataracts can all cause visual problems. The symptoms of different conditions can vary so make sure you keep up with your eye checks.

Some eye problems may be more serious than others and will require medical attention. Consult a doctor immediately if there is a sudden loss of vision or if everything appears hazy, even a temporary one. Call 911 or go straight to an emergency room.

Problems with Contact Lenses

These products work well for many people. However, you have to care for them. Make sure you wash your hands before touching them. Follow the instructions on how to use your medication. These rules should be followed:

You should never place them in your mouth. An infection may be more likely if you do this.

Make sure you have the correct fit for your lenses to ensure they don't scratch your eyes.

Make sure you only use eye drops that have a safety rating for contact lenses.

Use only professional saline solutions. While some lenses can be used to sleep with them, it is not FDA-approved.

If you're not sure if everything is correct but still have problems with your contacts, see your eye doctor. It could be that you have dry eyes, allergies, or just prefer glasses. Once you understand the issue, you can decide what solution is best for your needs.

Medicines for the Eyes

Chapter 2: Medicines And Food For The Eyes

Eye drugs are used for diagnosing, treating and preventing eye problems. Most eye medications need to be prescribed. OTC eye drops can be obtained as an over-the-counter option.

Eye drops and ointments are the most commonly used methods of treating the eye. Other delivery options include intravenous (tablets/capsules, liquids), intravenous ("shots"), and oral (tablets/capsules, liquids).

Why Eye Medications are necessary

Eye medications are commonly used to treat eye conditions such as glaucoma or eye infections. Eye drops can be used for diagnostic purposes, to dilate (enlarge), the pupils, or to color ocular surfaces in eye exams. Anesthetic eyedrops can be used to numb or dilate the eye. These are used to treat various conditions or to remove foreign matter from the cornea (the clear protective outer layer of your eye).

What is the correct use of eye meds?

It is important to know how to use eye drops.

Wash your hands.

You should shake the container.

Eye upwards and tilt your head.

Gently draw your lower eyelid away from the eyes, creating a pouch.

One drop, 1/4 to 1/2 inches of ointment should be added to the bag. You should not get in the eye with the container/dropper.

One of these methods can be used to make drops. Open your eyes and place your finger on either the inner corner of the eyelid or the side of the nose. This stops the drug from entering the tears duct and draining away.

Apply the ointment by closing your eyes. It is possible that your eyesight will be clouded for several moments.

If needed, repeat the procedure with the other eye.

Replace the cap or dropper from the bottle or tube and tighten.

It takes about five minutes for most eye drops to reach the eye. Do not introduce a second drop of eye drops or administer any other treatments without waiting at least five mins.

Some people have difficulty recognizing when they have correctly placed eye drops. Refrigerating the drops can improve the sensation of the drops reaching the eye.

Side effects of eye medications?

Side effects of eye drops

Eye drops could cause ocular adverse effects like redness, stinging and impaired vision. Eye infections can be caused by prolonged use of corticosteroids (e.g. Pred Forte or Decadron), a family of anti-inflammatory medicine called corticosteroids.

You should follow your ophthalmologist's instructions. In rare instances, some ocular decongestants (e.g. Visine and Murine Plus) can cause sudden (acute) glaucoma. If your eyes become red and painful after you use these drops, contact your eye doctor right away.

Anesthetic eye drop use can cause serious corneal damage. Anesthetic eyedrops can accidentally be given to injured eyes. This should not happen.

Eye problems can also be caused by drugs taken orally.

Side effects that can affect other parts of your body: Some eye drops could cause headaches or systemic side effect like diarrhea and stomach pains. Although the majority of systemic adverse effects that result from drops are minimal, serious reactions could occur. Beta-blocker medicine for glaucoma therapy (e.g. Timoptic Betagan or Betoptic), may cause adverse reactions.

These include lowering the heart rate and episodes of asthma, dropping blood pressure, confusion, memory loss, and loss sexual desire. Because these medicines may mask low blood sugar symptoms, diabetics should not take them.

Drops that dilate the pupils may cause pain during an eyecheckup. A few drops may cause dryness of skin and mouth, quick pulse, elevated heart rate, or high blood pressure in some individuals.

They can also cause more severe side effects, such as strokes and heart attacks in patients with high blood sugar, diabetes, and heart disease. Ophthalmologists can prevent these complications by taking a medical as well as an ocular history prior to performing an eye examination. You should inform your eye doctor if any of these conditions are present.

How can I avoid side effects?

Notifying your eye doctor or other physicians about any eye drops you take is essential. Many people forget to tell their doctor about their eye drops when they are asked by a nurse or doctor if they are taking prescriptions. Sometimes serious problems may arise when eyedrops are combined with another drug or with anesthesia. You should also inform your physician about any allergies.

With the use of multiple drops of eye medications, there is a greater chance of developing systemic adverse side effects. One-sixth as many eye drops can be stored in the eye than most commercial dropper bottle bottles. Excess medicine may either drop down the cheeks or drain into your nasolacrimal systems (the drainage mechanism for tears; please see figure).

Additional eye drops passing through the nasolacrimal systems can result in systemic adverse events. It is crucial to close your eye and push your finger into the corner of your eyes for five seconds before you add another drop.

Don't let children touch prescriptions. Intentionally ingesting eye drops can lead to serious adverse effects and death.

What's the Future for Eye Medicines in the Future?

Medical professionals are constantly looking for ways to minimize the side effects of eye medicines and make them more convenient and effective. New glaucoma medicine options are now available. These medicines minimize stinging, reduce the risk of systemic adverse effects and require fewer dosages each day. Researchers like the UIC Eye Center are looking at the benefits of using new treatments to treat the eye and seeking out improved ways to administer pharmaceuticals.

People believe that declining vision is inevitable as a result of age or eye strain. Healthy lifestyles can greatly reduce the risk of developing eye diseases.

Age-Related Eye Disease Study AREDS (2001) indicated that zinc, copper vitamin C, vitamin B, vitamin E and beta-carotene could lower the risk of eye health problems as we age.

This research was modified to test multiple versions of the original recipe in 2013. The variations included omega-3 fat acids, lutein, beta carotene, and zeaxanthin. However, some combinations may work better than other.

Further research shows that omega-3 oils (particularly DHA), copper as well as lutein and Zeaxanthin are vital for eye health.

This article will discuss the data supporting 10 nutritionally rich foods to promote good eye health. We will also examine eye health warnings and techniques to help healthy eyes.

Ten top eye-healthy foods

American Optometric Association, (AOA), as well as the American Academy of Ophthalmology, (AAO), continue to prescribe nutrition for good eye health based off the AREDS study.

The following 10 nutrient dense foods were supported by AREDS:

1. Fish

Eye disorders can be prevented by living a healthy lifestyle.

Many fish can provide omega-3 fatty oils.

Oily fish are those fish that have more oil in their bodies and stomachs. This makes them richer in omega-3 fish oil. The following fish are good sources of omega-3s:

tuna\salmon\strout\smackerel\sardines\anchovies\sherring

Studies have shown that fish oils can reverse dry eyes. This is especially true if you spend too much time at the computer.

2. Nuts & legumes

The omega-3 fatty acids found in nuts are also high. The high amount of vitamin E in nuts helps protect the eyes against age-related damage.

Most grocery shops sell nuts, and you can also buy them online. Eye-healthy legumes, and nuts, include:

Walnuts

Brazil nuts\cashews\peanuts\lentils\. Seeds

Like legumes and nuts, seeds are high-in omega-3s.

Most grocery stores and online retailers sell seed products. Seeds rich in omega-3 include:

chia seeds

Flax seeds Hemp seeds

4. Citrus fruits

Vitamin C is abundant in citrus fruits.

Citrus fruits high in vitamin C are:

lemons\oranges\grapefruits

5. Leafy green veggies

Leafy greens are high in lutein and Zeaxanthin. They also provide a strong source for eye-friendly vitamin D.

The most popular leafy greens are:

spinach\kale\collards

6. Carrots

Carrots are rich sources of Vitamin A and beta-carotene. Beta carotene gives carrots an orange hue.

Vitamin A plays an important role in the eyesight. Vitamin A is an essential component of the protein rhodopsin which allows light to be absorbed by the retina.

There is a lot of research into beta carotene and its effect on eyesight. The body requires this mineral in order to synthesize vitamin.

7. Sweet potatoes

Sweet potatoes have high levels of beta carotene just like carrots. They are also an excellent source of vitamin E.

8. Beef

Beef is high in zinc which has been linked for improved long-term eyesight. Zinc may prevent macular degeneration from occurring as a result of age-related vision impairment.

Zinc is found in high quantities in the eye's retina and the vascular tissues surrounding it.

Zinc is also present in meats such pig loin and chicken breast, though it is less than beef.

9. Eggs

Eggs are an excellent source of lutein as well as zeaxanthin. This may reduce the chance of developing age-related eye damage. The eggs are also rich in vitamin C, E, as well as zinc.

10. Water is essential to our eye health.

Drinking enough water can prevent dehydration. It may also reduce the symptoms of dry eye.

Daily intake recommended

The AAO recommends that you follow the AAO's current guidelines for eye health to prevent the development of eye disease.

500mg of vitamin C (400 international units)

10 mg lutein\s2 mg zeaxanthin\s80 mg of zinc oxide

2 milligrams Copper Oxide

Other eye health tips

Contact lenses wearers should always follow their doctors' instructions to minimize the risk of infection.

The AAO recommends the following practices for maintaining healthy eyes:

Avoid wearing sunglasses outside, as too much sun can cause cataracts. An online selection of sunglasses is available.

quitting smoking

Regular eye checks are recommended, particularly if there is a history of eye problems in the family.

Eye protection is recommended when dealing with eye irritants.

Before you place contacts, make sure to wash your hands.

Use contacts only for the duration suggested by the doctor or manufacturer\sprotecting eyes from computer-related eye strain by glancing away every 20 minutes at anything 20 feet away, for 20 seconds

Diabetes is the most common cause of blindness. People suffering from diabetes need to be vigilant about their blood sugar levels. They also need to take medication as directed by their doctor.

Early treatment can prevent eye problems from worsening. If you notice changes in your eyesight, it is a good idea to get an eye examination with either an optometrist/ophthalmologist.

Eye health indicators to watch out for

Signs that a person could be experiencing visual problems include:

Visual clarity fluctuates frequently

Viewing distorted images

Seeking flashes or floating objects in the field

diminished peripheral vision

Vitamin C, found in citrus fruits is thought to help lower the incidence of age-related retinal impairment.

To ensure good eye health, it is important to eat a diverse diet with plenty of fruits and vegetables.

People who are unable or unwilling to eat these nutrients should consult their eye doctor for eye health supplements.

A specialist should discuss the appropriate foods with people who have vision problems and those with restricted diets.

Chapter 3: Herbs That Improve Eye Sight

This might have happened because we live digitally. Let's take an in-depth look at the most important herbs for good eye health in 2022 that you and your staff can incorporate into their day.

1. Fennel

It was no accident that ancient Romans named fennel the "plant of sight". Vitamin A, Iron, along with minerals from this plant slow down cataract development and increase eyesight wellness.

How to Use it:

To make powder, grind 1 cup almonds with fennel and sugar.

To make a glass of milk, add a few teaspoons.

Drink before going to sleep.

Keep this program going for 40 days and you will see a change in your sight.

You might also like: 7 Effective Ways to Reduce Eye Strain in Work

2. Bilberry

It is rich in antioxidants called Anthocyanins. Similar compounds are found in blueberry (and cranberry), their botanical brothers. Royal Air Force pilots saw better in 1940s world war-II when they ate bilberry jelly.

Recent research has shown that bilberry does not have night vision enhancements, contrary to earlier research.

If you're an employee, it's a good healthy bet! Enjoy 50 gms bilberries as part of your lunch. The best results can be achieved by consuming it for several weeks.

We don't know if bilberry supplements can be used to help people with reduced night vision. One study indicated that anthocyanins (Ribes nigrum) from blackcurrants reduced eye fatigue, and also improved adaptation to the dark.

3. Green Tea

Free radicals cause so-called "oxidative damage". It is the cause of many chronic disorders such as cataracts and glaucoma. Green tea has antioxidants that absorb the free radicals.

In addition, laboratory studies show that the green tea's polyphenols can protect the retinal cell from UV radiation damage. UV radiation is a major cause of macular degeneration and cataracts.

You can make it every morning after you wake up. It might be possible to have it in your workplace with your lunch. It may help workers feel more awake and alert in the midst of monotonous job tasks.

4. Turmeric

Turmeric is a powerful antioxidant, and it's good for your eyes. Turmeric reduces the risk of eye oxidation. This results in the eye's clearness and precision.

Curcumin, another ingredient in turmeric, supports healthy eyes. Research has demonstrated that this chemical can be used to treat dry eyes.

It can also prevent the progression of retinal loss. Turmeric may be used to heal sore throats due to its anti-inflammatory abilities. This prevents the pharynx from becoming too irritated and allows for a more efficient functioning of the nose cavity.

For healthy eyes, workers should include turmeric into their daily diet.

5. Squash

The body can't make lutein, but squash supplies them throughout the year. Zinc and vitamin C are especially high in summer squash. The winter squash is also rich in omega-3 fat acids and vitamins A, C, and D.

Employers may make a mixed vegetable lunch by cooking a squash and vegetables.

This is a great way for employees to keep their appointment with an optometrist at bay.

6. Eyebright

Eyebright is a flower that can promote healthy eyes, which is quite strange considering its name. Eyebright has been proven to be effective in treating conjunctivitis. This is also known as pinkeye. It is highly contagious and can affect the health of workers at the workplace.

Blepharitis is an inflammation that occurs in the eyelids due to an eye infection. The eyebright could dramatically decrease inflammation and help to heal the condition.

It is possible to use this herb as a remedy for itchy, red eyes. Eyebright can also be used to treat the eyelids as a lotion. Eye drops that contain Eyebright extracts may also be available.

7. Ginkgo Biloba

It promotes blood circulation to the retina and soothes optic nerves. The retina is located in light-sensitive tissue near the back of the eyes. A preliminary study has shown that it may enhance the eyesight of patients with diabetes.

It is an antioxidant, which is particularly helpful for protecting nerve cell membranes, especially those in your eye.

8. Grapeseed

The grapeseed oil contains phytochemicals, which are good for the eyes. The extract also contains antioxidants as well as antihistamines. This enhances eye care.

Grapeseed extracts are now readily available commercially, so workers may consume them. The results could be evident in a few short weeks.

9. Indian Gooseberry (Amla) (Amla)

Ayurveda recognises amla as an effective remedy for improving eyesight. Amlas, also known by Indian gooseberries, are a great source of vitamin C.

Amla is rich in vitamin C which stimulates the activity and promotes healthy capillaries.

Add a few spoonfuls Amla juice to half of a cup of warm water. You can drink this twice daily, before bed and in the morning. Honey can be used to enhance the taste of amla.

10. Holy Basil (Tulsi),

Eye health concerns include irritation, infection, inflammation, and other inflammatory reactions that can lead poor eye health. Basil's antioxidants protect the eyes against oxidative damage and free radicals. Basil is not only effective at preventing eye problems, but it can also treat macular and cataract degeneration.

For employees to perform well at work, they must have the right eyesight. Workers must have regular eye examinations and be aware of the proper foods to ensure this happens.

Ingesting herbs that have shown to reduce visual problems will help you keep them away for the long-term. Take the time to get some herbs and try them out. Please let us know how these herbs make you feel.

Chapter 4: Exercises For The Eyes

Eye exercises have been advocated for years as a natural way to treat visual disorders. Eye exercises may improve your eyesight, but there isn't much scientific evidence to support this claim. Training your eyes may improve your eyesight and reduce eye strain.

Eye workouts will not be beneficial if you have an eye problem such as myopia, hyperopia, or astigmatism. Eye workouts won't be of any benefit to those with the most common eye disorders, including age-related Macular Degeneration, cataracts, and Glaucoma.

Eye exercises won't improve eyesight. However, they may help to relieve eye discomfort, especially if your eyes are irritated from work.

The problem of digital eye strain is common among computer users. This condition could cause:

Dry eyes = eye strainblurred sightheadaches

A few simple exercises could help with digital eye strain.

How to exercise eyes

Here are a few different types of eye workouts you could try depending on your need.

Focus on change

It works by increasing your concentration. This exercise should be performed from a sitting position.

Place your pointer fingers a few inches from your eyes.

Pay attention to your finger.

Slowly lift your finger from your face.

You can look out for a while into the faraway.

Your extended finger should be centered on your eyes.

Concentrate on the things in the distance and not your surroundings.

Do this three more times.

Near and distant focal points

This is another technique for concentration. This is another concentration practice. It should be done sitting down.

Tend your thumb approximately 10 inches in front of your face. Focus on it for 15 second.

Take a look at the item from 10-20 feet and then focus for 15 seconds.

Concentrate on your thumb.

Repeat the process five times.

Figure eight

It is best to do this exercise in a sitting position.

Focus on the area approximately 10 feet in front.

You can trace eight imagined figures with your eyes.

Keep following for 30 seconds. Then, swap directions.

20-20-20 rule.

Many people have eye strain. Our eyes are not meant to stay fixed on one thing for extended periods of time. The 20-20-20 rule could help to reduce digital eye strain if you work at a computer all the time. For this guideline to be applied, you should glance at everything 20 feet away once every 20 min.

What is vision therapy, exactly?

Vision therapy is a specialization of some physicians. Vision therapy may include exercises for the eyes, but only when it is part of a larger treatment plan that is overseen by an eye doctor or optometrist.

Vision therapy can be used to strengthen your eye muscles. It may also assist with the correction of poor visual behavior and eye tracking disorders. Vision therapy may be helpful for both children and adults.

Convergence Insufficiency

strabismus (cross-eye or walleye) (cross-eye or walleye)

amblyopia (lazy eye) (lazy eye)

Dyslexia

Tips for improving your eye health

You can do many things to keep your eyes healthy.

A complete dilated exam of the eyes should be performed every couple years. Get a test even if you haven't detected difficulties. Many people don't realize that they may be able to see better with corrective sunglasses. Many eye disorders are not easily diagnosed.

Get to know your family history. Many eye issues are genetic.

Know your risk. Eye problems are more common in people with diabetes and those who have a history of eye disease. Make sure to see your eye doctor at least six months out.

Wear sunglasses. Protect your eyes with polarized sunglasses. They filter out both UVA & UVB radiation.

Healthily eat. Healthy diets rich in antioxidants and healthy fats may be beneficial for your eyes. Eat those carrots! They are a fantastic source of vitamin-A, which is vital for eye health.

Contact lenses or glasses may be required if you have vision impairments. Corrective glasses won't cause your eyes to be weaker.

Smoking is a terrible habit that can be difficult to quit. Smoking is harmful for your entire body and eyes.

Eye workouts have not been shown to improve people's vision. Eye workouts may not be able to help, but they aren't likely to cause damage. Regular eye exams by an eye doctor are essential. They are often able to identify and correct problems before any symptoms become apparent.

Three Eye Exercises for Strabismus Relief

What is Strabismus?

Strabismus is commonly referred to as "crossed eyes", but it can also be called crossed eyes. The American Optometric Association defines strabismus "a condition where both eyes cannot stare in the exact same spot at the time." This might be manifested as one eye sliding inward or forth (exotropia), upwards (hypertropia), downwards (hypotropia), or in between (esotropia). This is usually due to incongruities. For example, the eye may not be able to focus properly on a distant point.

Strabismus occurs most often in infants and toddlers. This can be due to genetics or other issues that arise during physical development. Many cases of Strabismus in young people are caused by poor communication between brain, muscles, or nerves. It may also happen in those who have had a stroke, brain injury, or diabetes. If untreated, this issue can cause double vision, loss or diminished depth awareness, as well as possible loss of sight.

What are the treatments for strabismus?

Treatments range from prescription glasses to surgery to align the eye. Many vision rehabilitation programs include exercises for the eyes. These could help with coordination.

You should not treat exercises as a treatment for diseases. Dr. Jeffrey Anshel founded the Ocular Nutrition Society.

"Because there are many causes and presentations of strabismus, patient driven eye exercises should not alone be treated." "An optometrist and orthoptist can properly diagnose the condition, and recommend a treatment regimen that targets specific symptoms."

Before beginning any vision therapy, it is important to have an eye exam.

Pencil pushups

Pencil pushing ups are a basic ocular exercise that helps both eyes to focus in the same spot. They are also known to be called near point convergence exercises.

Start by holding a pencil straight out in front of you. Concentrate your attention on the eraser or the letter or number at the side. Slowly drag the pencil towards your nose. It is important to keep it focused for as long and as possible. However, if you have blurred vision, stop.

Brock string

Frederick Brock, a Swiss optometrist devised the practice to improve eye coordination. A string about 5 feet long will be required with three different colored beads.

You can attach one end to a fixed spot such as a railing. Space the beads evenly. The string's other end should be kept close to your nose.

When moving your gaze from one to the next, you should be able to see a constant pattern. The bead will become visible by itself when it reaches the junction of two strings that are identical to each other. If you see the strings crossing in the front or back of the beads, your eyes might not be correctly focused. All beads must have an X (except for one at the far edge, where the two threads will be coming towards you in a V).

Move the beads along the thread to reposition them and then resume the practice.

Barrel cards

This is an excellent practice for exotropia. On one side, draw three barrels increasing in size in length in red. Do the exact same thing in reverse.

To find the closest barrel, hold the card horizontally and vertically. Stare at the distant bar until you have a picture of both the colors and two other images.

Keep your eyes fixed for at least five seconds. Repeat the process with the smaller and middle barrel images.

Chapter 5: You Can Test Your Eyesight

A visual ability test (or vision acuity) is an eye examination that tests how well you are able to perceive details of letters or symbols from a certain distance.

Visual acuity describes your ability recognize the details and forms in the objects you see. This is only one aspect your whole eyesight. There are also color vision, peripheral and depth vision.

There are many forms of visual impairment tests. The majority of these are basic. Depending on the type of exam and the location it was administered, the exam could be:

An optometrist is an opticiansan opticiansa techniciansa nursing

There are no hazards in visual acuity test, and there's no need for any preparation.

Scope of the exam

If you feel your vision is blurred or you have difficulty seeing, an eye exam might be necessary. A full eye exam includes more than just the visual acuity tests.

A routine visual acuity exam is performed on all children. Early diagnosis and evaluation of visual disorders could help to prevent future problems.

Optometrists, drivers license bureaus, among other organizations use this exam to verify your eyesight.

How the visual-acuity test works

Snellen is a widely-used test, as well as random E.

Snellen

The Snellen Test uses a chart that lists symbols and letters. The chart was undoubtedly displayed in an eye doctor or school nurse office. The letters are different sizes and are organized in rows or columns. This chart is visible from a distance of 14 to

20 feet. It helps determine your ability read letters and forms.

During the exam your eyes will be covered by one eye and you'll either stand or sit at a distance from the chart. Your uncovered eye will allow you to read the letters aloud. The same process will be repeated for your second eye. Your doctor may recommend that you start to read smaller letters until it becomes difficult to distinguish letters.

Random E

In the random E Test, you will find out which direction letter "E" is facing. The direction that the letter faces will be determined by looking at it on a chart or projection.

These tests are often more complicated when they are performed in an optometrist's office than in a nurses office. A mirror reflection of the chart can also be displayed at an eye clinic. The chart will be seen through many different lenses. Your doctor will replace the lenses until you can see the chart clearly. If you require vision correction, your doctor will swap out the lenses until you can read the chart clearly.

Understanding your test results

Visual acuity may be described as a fraction, like 20/20. 20/20 vision means your visual acuity at 20ft from an object is normal. To see an object, you will need to be 20ft away if you have 20/40 sight. This is a difference from what people can see from 40ft away.

Corrective eyeglasses or contact lenses may be necessary if your vision isn't 20/20. A possible eye disease, such an infection or damage, should also be addressed. Your doctor will review your results with you and discuss any therapy or corrections.

Here's an overview of all the possible tests your eye doctor may run during an eye examination.

Applanation Tonometry

This test measures how much pressure it takes for a cornea section to be flattened. Your doctor can measure pressure to detect and keep track of glaucoma. They will first give drops to numb you eye. Then, they will use a tonometer to gently touch it.

Corneal Topography

The cornea's curvature is measured by an automated examination. This could indicate abnormalities on your eye's cornea, such as scarring, swelling, disease, or conditions like astigmatism. It can be seen before you have surgery, a transplant of the cornea, or a fitting for contact lenses.

Fluorescein Angiogram

This allows doctors to see how blood flows through your retina. It is useful in diagnosing diabetic retinopathy and retina detachment. Fluorescein, a special dye, will be injected into your veins. It quickly reaches the blood vessels inside your eye. The doctor then uses a camera equipped with special filters to highlight the dye. They photograph the dye as it passes through your blood vessels. This allows them to identify blood vessel abnormalities, swelling, leakage, and circulation disorders.

Exam of the Dilated Pepillary

This is what the doctor uses to stretch your eye's pupil. This allows them inspect your retina to detect signs of illness.

Refraction

This is how your doctor will obtain your prescription for eyeglasses. You look at a chart from about 20 feet away or in a mirror which makes it seem like you're only 20 feet away. A phoropter allows you to look through a handheld device. It allows doctors to adjust different strengths of lenses right in front of your eyes. You might tell them if objects look clear or fuzzy. Your answers give them your prescription to your contact lenses and glasses. You will also find out if you have presbyopia (hyperopia), myopia (myopia), and astigmatism.

Slit-Lamp Study

The microscope is used to shine a light beam on your eye that is shaped like an opening in the eye. During the examination, they may dilate your pupils. It can be used to diagnose cataracts, glaucoma and detached retinas.

Non-Contact Tonometry

This test helps to identify glaucoma. The doctor will use a device called a "tonometer" to blow a small amount of air. This measure indirect ocular pressure through the response to the air.

An applanation instrument may also measure pressure. Although they are the most precise, you will still need local anesthesia.

Retinal Tomography

This computerized examination might provide a clear view of all layers of the retina. This examination could be done if there is a significant retina problem like age-related retinal degeneration or retinal dislocation.

Ultrasound

This test uses sound waves in order to obtain an image of your inner eye. It can help your doctor detect and treat cataracts, tumors, or bleeding within your eye. It is also possible to get it before cataract surgery.

Visual Acuity Testing

This tests your ability to see well at both local and long distances. A test is conducted if the youngster cannot read. Your youngster will need to be able to see the letter "E" with his/her eyes and then show the doctor where the legs point. Before the exam, you can practice this at home.

Visual Field Test

This test will evaluate your peripheral (side), eyesight. An object will be placed in the middle or near the center of your field of vision. As you gaze at the target, note whether or not you see an object moving within your visual field. This test can help the doctor determine if you have been suffering from eye diseases such as stroke and glaucoma.

Chapter 6: Eyesight Improvement Myths Busted

"We barely know how much pleasure and interest we get in life through our eyes. Until then, we can't do without them. But part of that pleasure is the fact that the eyes are able to choose where they want to look. "But the ears can't decide where to listen," Ursula K. Le Guin

Most people would agree that their eyes make life more interesting, brighter and more colorful. Unfortunately, people have misguided many others in human society by telling people things that aren't true. What about eating an absurd amount of carrots or raw spinach?

So, here are top myths regarding improving eyesight - all busted!

Avoid too close to your TV. It will cause you to lose your vision! BUSTED

Many people, including some doctors, agree that too much television is damaging to your eyes. Let's not forget that this is not supported by any scientific evidence. Dr. Lee Duffner MD claims that people can choose where they feel most comfortable.

When a person sits too close in front of a TV, or in a room with low lighting, the eyes can get tired. It is easy to get tired of the TV. It doesn't mean you can all be glued to the TV. Eye fatigue can cause strain to the eyes, and even severe headaches.

You can't read in dark places dear. BUSTED

This is something many people have heard often. Many people read books before they go to sleep. Dr. Harvey Moscot of Healthy Magazine said that reading in dark places, much like watching TV, is tiring on the eyes. While it won't alter your vision, it could cause eye fatigue. To prevent eye-fatigue, it is a good idea to keep a lamp lit at night so you can read. Eye fatigue can cause severe headaches and strain the eyes.

Eye health is improved by eating lots of spinach and carrots. BUSTED

This is a myth. You don't need to eat spinach or carrots like a rabbit to see like an animal! Some people have vision problems even though they eat carrots for breakfast and lunch. A diet high in carrots is not healthy. To get the best results, limit the intake of tomatoes, spinach, tomatoes, oranges and other vegetables. It's also true that carrots contain vitamin B which is great to have for a healthy diet.

LASIK eye operations can cure vision. BUSTED

This isn't a permanent solution. It is possible to require a repeat treatment. You should discuss any follow-up treatments with your doctor if you're seriously considering LASIK.

Blindness can be caused from excessive sex, masturbation, and genital sex - BUSTED

This is false. Everyone can enjoy sex without being blind. Half the world would be blind if this was true. Then, people would be afraid of discussing their sex lives. One can become blind if they have a sexually transmitted infection like Syphilis.

After you reach 40, it is a good idea to have your eyes checked regularly. BUSTED

Even if one has no vision issues, it doesn't matter. No matter your age, it's recommended that you have your eyes examined regularly. It is possible to treat any condition if you get it diagnosed early. Many eye conditions can now be treated thanks to medical advancements. Glaucoma is one example of a condition that can affect anyone before 40.

It's possible to have an entire eye transplanted by doctors! BUSTED

This is not possible. It is impossible for any doctor to transplant an entire eye. The eyes are connected with the brain's optical nerve. If you want to have an entire eye transplant, your eye must be connected. We are not machines that can open, unplug and plug things. Although medical science has come a long way, it is still far from the extent that it was in the past. Part eye transplant differs from full eye surgery. Only certain parts of an eye are replaced.

Only look at the sun with your sunglasses on - BUSTED

The sun's ultraviolet lights can be extremely strong regardless of whether one is wearing sunglasses. It can cause temporary vision impairment, headaches, and can even damage sensitive eye parts. You should be aware that even if you have sunglasses on, direct sunlight can blind you in as little a half an minute.

Chapter 7: Eye-Friendly Foods

This is not about eating carrots, spinach, and treating it as if you were a wild graminivore! Most people will be able to agree with the following.

It's not just about eating carrots.

Keep in mind that eye-friendly diets are not quick fixes and won't (in fact, nothing will) cure you overnight. It may take years for your vision to turn to unhealthy eating habits. Understanding that it is possible to reverse the effects of these changes, you will need to alter certain ingrained patterns that you have acquired over the years. This book contains exercises that will help to reverse the damage already done.

Foods to Support Your Eyes

There are many healthy food options that you can choose to help your eyesight and to make it easier to live a more balanced life. These foods can help people see better. It can be dangerous to eat only one type of food like spinach and carrots. This will cause your body to lack essential minerals and vitamins it needs to perform its functions. For the health of your whole body, it's important to eat a variety healthy foods. Note that omega-rich fish is good for eyes and the whole body. You will reap the benefits of the following foods, however, you need to make sure that there is no excess oil, other than olive oil, when cooking them for breakfast, lunch and dinner.

Fruits

Dried Apricots

Cnataloupe

Persimmons

Guava

Blueberry

Lemon

Kiwi Fruit

Barbados Cherry

Bilberry

Vegetables

Broccoli

Celery

Green Beans

Peas

Brussels Sprouts

Corn

Tomatoes

Carrots

Sweet Pepper

Chili Peppers

Collards

Leaf Lettuce

Dandelion Leaves

Spinach

Leeks

Mustard Leaves

Squash

Kale

Sweet Potatoes

Yam

Fish

Sardine

Salmon

Mackerel

Albacore Tuna

These foods are easy to add to your daily diet. So, if you've had a carrot salad for breakfast, you might want sweet potatoes for lunch. Or, you may have sweet potato salad for breakfast. In order to make your body healthier, it is important to choose the foods you enjoy eating.

There are certain foods you should avoid.

Keep your eyes open.

It is best to avoid eating too many red meats and junk food, as they can be harmful for your eyes and health.

Why? Many chemicals, oils, and large amounts of sugar are used in the production of these foods. This makes them difficult to digest and hinders the body's ability to benefit. They might taste great; who doesn't like donuts, cream bagels, and other delicious foods? But these seemingly delicious, flavor-enhancing foods don't have anything to offer other than fats and cholesterol.

It is important to avoid excessive salt intake as this could lead to other health problems.

These are some of the delicious recipes that include key ingredients.

Maple-Mustard Glaze Roasted Salmon

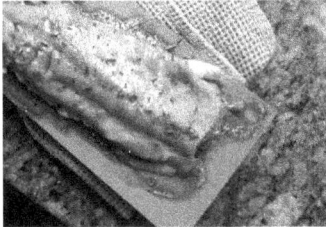

Ingredient List:

For 2 or more people:

1 and a 1/2 pounds de-boned salmon filet

2 tablespoons of whole grain mustard

2 teaspoons maple sugar

Salt and fresh ground black pepper are two of the best ways to make your taste buds stand out

Lemon wedges as garnish

Directions:

Preheat oven to 475o Farenheight

Rinse and pat dry the fish. Place the fish skin side down on parchment-lined baking sheets. (The parchment prevents the fish sticking to the pan, and significantly reduces cleanup.

In the salmon, make a half-inch crosshatch. Season lightly with salt and pepper.

Mix the maple syrup with the mustard. Apply the mustard to the fish. Bake on the middle rack of your oven for 10-12 mins or until salmon is cooked through. Take the salmon out of oven. To complete the cooking process, cover it with foil. Serve with a squeeze of lime.

California Tuna Sandwiches

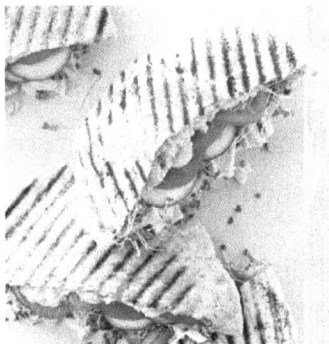

Ingredient List:

3/4 cup Guacamole

6 oz (1 can) albacore tuna, drained

1 1/2 cups celery, diced

1 1/2 cups onion diced

6 pita pocket bread

6 leaves romaine lettuce

1/4 cup Radishes, chopped

Directions:

If you do not have a prepared variety of guacamole, make it according to the recipe.

Combine the guacamole (tuna, celery and onion) in a bowl and mix well.

Lightly toast pita bread pockets and then cut in half. Half of the tuna mixture should be stuffed into each half.

Garnish the dish with radish slices

Recipe courtesy on recipe wikia

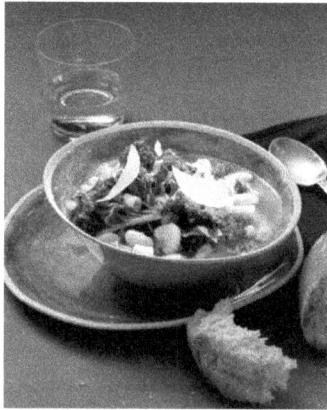

Soup of Kale and Beans

Ingredient List:

1 tbsp olive oil/canola oil

6-8 cloves of minced garlic

1 large onion, chopped

4 cups chopped kale if fresh. If frozen, you can freeze 2 or 3 pkgs. Use 2 to 3 cans of canned kale

4 cups of vegetable or chicken broth

2 x 15oz cans white beans of any variety

1 can of diced fresh tomatoes or stewed tomato sauce

1 tsp dried rosemary

1 tsp rosemary

Salt and pepper to suit your taste

1 cup chopped Parsley

Directions:

In a large pan, heat olive oil and then add garlic to the pot.

Mix these ingredients together until smooth.

Add the kale to the pan and cook until tender.

3. Cups of broth, 2 cups of beans and tomatoes. Add herbs, salt, pepper, and other seasonings.

Let sit for 5-10 minutes.

Blend the remaining beans with the broth in a blender until smooth. It's to thicken it, I bet you are asking.

Make soup.

Allow to sit for 15 to 20 seconds.

Serve it up in bowls with parsley.

Recipe courtesy of Portuguese-recipes.com

Eye Friendly Juices

This isn't your regular juice you make with milk and water. Each of the listed juices must have at the least one of these essential ingredients and the desired ingredient, depending on what condition the person is in.

An additional ingredient may be added to the juice. The essential ingredient must be present in at least 50% to 75%. To make up the balance, the rest of the ingredients can be added. Make sure to keep the juice refrigerated for future thawing.

Take the ingredients and blend them in a blender. It will take some effort to blend slowly, but the result will be rich in vitamins and nutrients - all the body needs for good health.

Essential Ingredients

Broccoli

Chard Dandelion

Kale

Parsley

Spinach

Watercress

Best's Disease: Don't eat too much fruit

Apples

Grapes

Raspberries

Beets

Cabbage

Carrots

Celery leeks

Spinach

Ginger

Garlic

Parsley

Lemon

Chlorophyll

Wheat Grass

Conjunctivitis, Cataracts

Apple

Blueberry

Carrot

Celery

Endive

Spinach

Parsley

Macular Deterioration

Broccoli

Green Bell Pepper

Greens

Red Bell Pepper

Apples

Raspberries

Floaters

Apples

Raspberries

Beets

Carrots

Celery

Parsnip

Garlic Parsley

Optic Nerve Problems

Chlorophyll

Wheat Grass

Berries

Beets

Cabbage

Carrots

Endive

Ginger

Diabetic Retinopathy

Raspberries

Ginger

Garlic

Parsley

Chlorophyll

Artichokes

Asparagus

Beets

Cabbage

Carrots

Celery

Leeks

Pumpkin

Spinach

Glaucoma

Raspberries

Plums

Apples

Turnips

Radish

Parsley

Cucumber

Celery

Carrots

Cabbage

Beets

Retinitis Pigmentosis (don't use too much fruits)

Grapes

Raspberries

Lemon

Chlorophyll

Wheat Grass

Ginger

Garlic Beets

Cabbage

Carrots

Celery

Leeks

Parsley

Spinach

Foods to Keep at a Minimum

French fries, chicken fried steak and all other types of fried food are included. Blood vessels are a part of our eyes and need to be cared for just as with the rest. You would not want fat deposits in your eyes to clog your arteries.

Get drunk on alcoholic beverages This can cause permanent blurred vision or double-vision. Moderate drinking i.e. Moderate drinking is 1 glass for women and 2 glasses for men.

The Nicotine products include cigarettes, cigars and tobacco. You are at greater risk of developing cataracts, dry vision and macular disease. You can quit using nicotine products.

Red meats, such as lamb, pork, or beef. Saturated fats as well as cholesterol can buildup in the macular vessels, slowing down blood flow. Moderation is key. You should eat less than 4 times per week

This includes processed meats such as bacon, sausages or luncheon and dinner meats. Consuming a lot of these foods, as well as red meats, can cause macular disease. You should eat in moderation. You should eat less than 4 times per week

Baked goods that contain cream dripping cake, pastries and cookies, as well as donuts and any other sugary treats. Please eat moderation. Eat less than 2 times per week

Excessive oil intake. This is bad for your eyes and body. As much as possible, reduce it.

Chapter 8: Herbs That Improve Vision Naturally

Additional information is available about herbs that improve natural vision.

Spices & Herbs

Turmeric

Oregano

Dill

Parsley

Aspalathus

Bilberry

Passion Flower

Gingko

Biloba

Bilwa

Mahonia

Grape

Golden Seal

These herbs are easily found at the local grocery store, or in an herbal shop. Like all other types of medicine before trying any type of herbal treatment, it is important to consult a qualified herbalist.

Aspalathus

This herb is a South African native and is sometimes called Rooibos. It is a powerful herb, and its properties are very similar to bilberries. This herb contains antioxidants that can help improve the overall health and immune system.

Bilberry

Because they contain bioflavonoids (a powerful element that reduces macular deterioration), this herb is mainly used in therapeutic treatment. This herb can prevent the development of any retinal diseases and protect the veins and blood vessels from further damage. It is possible to significantly improve your vision clarity and distance-seeing ability by using this herb. It also improves nightvision. It will not benefit those who are short-sighted, farsighted, or have cataracts.

Passion Flower

This herb is said to help relax the blood vessels of the eyes and ease eye strain due to constant focus on objects or excessive reading in dim areas.

Gingko Biloba

This herb can increase blood flow to eyes. Macular degeneration sufferers can benefit from this herb's ability to prevent retinal damage.

Bilwa

This herb is great if you have sties and frequent conjunctivitis.

Mahonia Grape Extracts

This herb can help protect sensitive eyes from the harmful effects of the sun's ultraviolet rays. It protects your eyes from the damaging UV rays from the sun. It also strengthens your eye's capillaries and maintains eye health.

Golden Seal

This herb is known to have soothing properties. It soothes eyes when the eyes become irritated, inflamed, or otherwise damaged. This herb is a great choice for those who need some pain relief.

Chapter 9: How Medical Drugs Can Damage Your Eyes

Certain medical conditions require that people take prescribed medicine every day. The problem is that some medicines can cause permanent damage to the eyes.

This is a common misconception. They aren't aware of this fact, so they don't ask the doctor if prescribed medications could cause any eye damage. Make sure you ask your doctor for information about any possible eye problems. Google is a great way to research any medication you are prescribed. Although these medications have been shown to cause damage to the eyes, not everyone is affected. Ask your doctor for clarification.

Steroids

If you are taking steroids, talk to your doctor about replacing the steroid treatment by natural cortisone. To minimize the negative effects on your eyes, make sure to include vitamin E or C in your daily diet.

Eye Hemorrhage: Drugs that Can Cause Eye Hemorrhage

* Venlafaxine, an antidepressant

* Pentoxifylline- a drug that is commonly used to prevent blood clotting

* Non-Steroidal Anti-Inflammatory Drugs,

* Some over-the counter drugs

* Amphotericin B- An antibiotic

* Oral anticoagulants for Heparin and Anisidione such as Coumadine or Coumadine.

* Cholesterase inhibitors – Used to treat Alzheimer's.

Cornea Treatments

These drugs can make the cornea change, which can lead to halos around light. They can also increase light and glare sensitivities and reduce visual clarity. The symptoms might disappear as soon as the medication is stopped. This is common for some people. Ask your doctor if this would cause any harm.

* Quinacrine,

* Hydroxychloroquine,

* Chloroquine.

Drugs that may cause macular deterioration and/or cataracts

* Birth Control Pills

* Sulfa drugs

* Antihistamines,

* Antidepressants/Tranquilizers

* Steroids,

* Oral antidiabetic drugs

* Antibiotics, including Fluroquinone Mefloquine or Terbinafine

* Prednisone,

* Advil. Advil. Apsirin. Meclofen.

* Isoretinoin or Eretinate

Drugs That May Damage the Retina

* Clonidine is also known as Catapres. It's used to lower blood Pressure.

Plaquenil - A drug that is prescribed to patients suffering from rheumatoidarthritis.

* Thioridazine,

* Tylenol. Ketoprofen. Flurbiprofen. Aspirin. Naproxen Sodium. Ibuprofen. Aleve. Bayer. Montrin.

Drugs that Can Reduce Blood Flow To The Eyes

* Estrogen,

* The synthetic hormones androgen replacements

Drugs that Can Cause Glaucoma or Damage to the Optic Nerve

* Venlafaxine,

* Fenfluramine,

* Antidepressants

* Steroids (like Presnisone),

* Mitazapine,

* Simvastatin,

* Gastric Antispasmodics

* NSAID medications.

Although people often resort to these drugs to ease pain and discomfort, many don't realize the dangers it could cause to their eyes. Ask your doctor if there are any safer options. The battle is only half won if your eyes are saved from irreparable damage.

Chapter 10: Natural Eye Exercises To Improve Vision

The importance of maintaining good eyesight is often stressed. It is vital to eat right foods and to practice eye exercises in order to keep your vision clear. This will help prevent you from becoming blind at any age. Most people discover that glasses or contact lens are not necessary in order to see well. Some try to reverse the effects. Others continue to flow with the process and some eventually become blind in their golden years.

However, people often believe that once your vision is poor, there is nothing you can do to fix it. This book will explain how to improve vision naturally. It is important to try the exercises one at time. It's unrealistic to expect immediate results. It takes time. These exercises cannot be used to replace medical advice. Your doctor should be consulted before you begin any eye exercise.

Exercise 1 - Improve Focus

This exercise will improve your focus ability. This exercise should be repeated 10 times per day. If you do this regularly, you will achieve significant results.

Step 1

Make sure the object is no more than three feet from you. Look closely at the object until it is clearly identified.

Step 2

Once Step 1 has been completed, you can now look at objects placed closer to your eyes. It is important to look at it closely, so that all its features and attributes are clearly identifiable.

Step 3

Take a look at objects located 500 feet away. It is important to look closely at each object, so that all its aspects and features are easily identified.

Step 4

Take a look at objects that are far away. It is important to look at it closely without getting too close. When all its features have been identified, move the eye to the nearest object.

Exercise 2 Distance viewing

This is the perfect exercise to enhance your distant viewing abilities.

Step 1

Place the pencil or finger in front your face, about an arm's reach. Keep your left eye closed and keep your right eye open.

Step 2

Now, open your left eyes and look as far away as you can.

Step 3

Now, focus with your left eye on the pencil/finger and bring back the vision to the finger/pencil that is in front.

Step 4

Now open your right ear and focus as far as you can. You can repeat Steps 1 and 4 up to 20 to 30 more times.

Exercise 3 - Increase Blood Circulation to Your Eyes

This exercise will strengthen neck muscles which in turn will increase blood flow and oxygen to the head and eyes. The exercise requires that the person move their head up or down. To ensure safety, it is best to do this slowly and carefully.

Step 1

Place your head straighten and relax.

Step 2

Now, tilt your head backwards so that you can see the ceiling or sky. Keep this position for a few moments.

Step 3

Now, move your head downwards like you're trying to see the ground. Keep this position for a few seconds.

Step 4

To achieve significant results, go back to step 1. Repeat this process 10 times daily.

Exercise 4 – Eye Muscle development and increased flexibility

This exercise will increase flexibility, as well as strengthen the muscles surrounding the eyes.

Step 1

Imagine a giant 8-pointed figure positioned just 10 feet from your eyes.

Step 2

Use a little imagination to turn this massive figure 8 on its side.

Step 3

Calm your mind and let it go. The outline of the gigantic figure 8 can be traced slowly and clockwise using your eyes.

Step 4

Once the figure is complete, trace it clockwise. After that, let your eyes relax. Do this four times daily.

Exercise 5: To Relieve Eye Pressure (Amazing for computer users)

This exercise is great for both people who are always on their computer and those who just want to ease eye stress. You will get the best results by doing this exercise as often and frequently as you can.

Step 1

Relax in a comfortable place and remove any contact lenses or glasses. Take a few deep inhalations.

Step 2

For heat, place your elbows on a table.

Step 3

After some heat has been generated in the palms close your eyes and place your palms over the eyes. Place the palms over the eyes without putting pressure. You should still be able to blink even after placing them on your eyes. Cover your eyes with the palms and keep them covered for around 15 minutes.

Step 4

Look around and notice if the colors are brighter. Do objects seem sharper? Can you see more clearly with your glasses on? If so, don't stop working with your glasses. It will take a while for the eyes back to the normal state. This exercise will take longer to bring the eyes back to normal, but you will notice improvements each time.

Chapter 11: Tips For Improving Your Night Vision

Would you like to be able to see well in the dark? Although it is possible, you must be patient as there are no quick fixes. Let's begin by stating the following:

1. Avoid bright light - it takes approximately 30 minutes for the eyes adjust to darkness. Also, glaring at bright lights can slow the process.

2. Utilize peripheral vision. This means that you can look at all of the objects simultaneously and not just one.

3. You should move your eyes frequently, rather than focusing on an object for prolonged periods of times.

4. Because humans are nearly color-blind, look out for shapes, lines, and movement in the dark.

5. A person who is suddenly required to see outside in the daylight should close one eye.

6. Instead of looking at a source lamp, see what's below it. Instead of looking at a streetlamp or pole, focus on the pole.

7. Your blood sugar levels also affect night vision. Retina and the cells of the brain need glucose to enable them to see in the dark. Take a sugar cube or a few dried cherries, plums, or raw plums.

Chapter 12: Vision And Choosing The

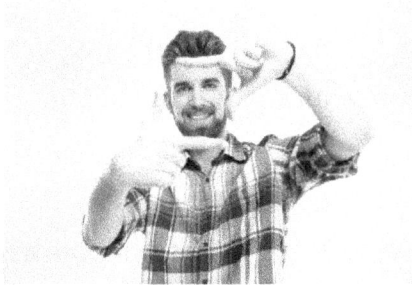

Natural Way

The majority of people who wear prescription glasses do not like wearing them. Contact lenses are not suitable for everyone. If there is one thing we know about eye vision it is that everyone wants to have clearer eyesight.

The truth is, there are alternatives to prescription glasses and contacts for better vision. Furthermore, you don't have to use prescription glasses to see clearly.

Do not misunderstand me. Prescription glasses serve a purpose. They can assist the eyes in dealing with certain conditions that have been diagnosed. Sometimes, the only option is to put them on. It is possible to have your eyes corrected by surgery.

However, there are problems when one relies on advanced methods to improve his eyesight (e.g. surgery) are diverse. These are certainly more expensive than the natural way to achieve better vision. You will spend a lot of money on contacts and eyeglasses, especially if you go to reputable shops that are well-respected for quality products. There is no way you can just pick up any pair of non-prescription glasses on the street, believing that this will suffice to alleviate your problems. A number of eye conditions can make it necessary to regularly change prescription glasses due to deteriorating vision. This is not only annoying, but can also lead to high costs.

Additionally, surgery can pose serious medical risks. These procedures can cause serious eye injuries, including corneal scarring, infection, and ruptures.

It is important to understand that you don't have to suffer from the discomfort of wearing eyeglasses. You may also be unable to afford or unwilling to go under the needle for eye surgery. There are other options, which this book will explain in the next chapters.

Natural eyecare is something that everyone can do. It doesn't require a specific age, ethnicity, or socioeconomic status. The added benefit is that natural things you do to improve your vision can have a positive impact on your whole body.

If you are open to natural methods of improving your sight, you will enjoy lower medical costs, a healthier body and better vision.

Chapter 13: Parts Of Your Eye And The

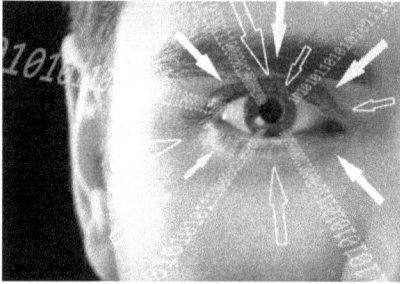

Visual Process

The eye, one of our most sensitive organs, is involved in many complex processes. Understanding how your eyes work will allow you to better understand the various eye conditions. This chapter will provide detailed information about vision.

1. Cornea

The cornea is the outer coating of the eye that protects it and its inner parts from the elements. Your cornea will eventually become damaged and you will lose your sight.

2. Sclera

This refers the whites of your eye and is responsible to provide structure and safety for inner components of your eye.

3. Pupil

The pupil is the small black dot that lies in the middle of your eye. A hole allows light to pass through so your eyes can focus properly on any object in its path.

4. Iris

Your eyes' color comes from your iris. The uniqueness of the iris is what gives us our eyes their color. It contains pigments that determine whether we will have emerald or brown eyes. Another function of iris is the ability to take in more or less sunlight depending on your surroundings. This means it is responsible for both dilation (when your pupil looks larger) and contraction.

5. Conjunctiva Glands

These layers of mucus keep your eyes' outside moist.

6. Lacrimal glands

This area of the eye is responsible to produce tears that help moisturize the eye. In the outer corner of each eyes are the lacrimal cells.

7. Retina

The retina, which is located at the back end of the eye's eyes, is an integral component of the visual systems. It is composed of rods, cones, and chemical components that transform light into electrical impulses and chemicals that can be interpreted by the brain. It is also directly connected with the optic nerve.

8. Choroid

This area of the eye is between the retina (sclera) and the retina. It supplies blood to your eyes.

9. Vitreous Humor

The vitreous Humor is a gel in the back that keeps the eye's shape in place.

10. Aqueous Humor

The aqueous Humor, on the other side, is a watery substance, which fills your eyes.

11. Lens

The lens is a layer of clear material that lies directly behind your pupil. It helps to reflect light back into the cornea. It also focuses light that is absorbed by it. It can adjust its form to enable the eyes, which are able to see objects from different distances, a phenomenon known as accommodation.

Accommodation is achieved by bringing in both near- and far stimuli under one roof. The lens will flatten if the stimuli at a distance and bulge if it is close.

The visual process begins when light, reflected by stimuli (e.g. Through your pupil, light from the stimuli (e.g. tree or other person) enters your retina. Your lens, which focuses the light through your cornea to sharpen the retina's image of the stimuli, helps you focus it. The retina includes the rods as well as the cones. These visual receptors contain chemicals called "visual pigments" that are sensitive to light. These visual pigments react to light reflected from stimuli, triggering electrical impulses. These electrical signals are sent from the retina to the optic nervous, which conducts them towards the brain.

Chapter 14: Eye Conditions To Watch For

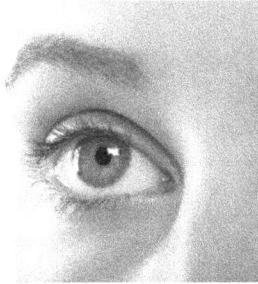

The eye can become a vulnerable part in our bodies, especially when the defense mechanisms that were designed to protect it fail. The eye can develop many diseases and conditions that can affect vision and cause total blindness. These conditions can develop from a variety factors including genetics and environmental factors. We will be discussing some of the most common conditions in the eye. Some eye problems are the result of poor preventive measures. Others are caused by our lifestyles and bodily changes such as aging. It is important that you take note of these eye conditions to understand what can happen and how to prevent them.

1. Viral conjunctivitis

Also known as pinkeye, this eye problem can cause reddening of the whites of your eyes due to an infection in your eye's conjunctiva. This condition can also be brought on by allergic reactions and other physical agents.

The conjunctiva covers your eyeballs and lines your eyelids. This eye condition can be very common as the conjunctiva has to constantly be exposed to microorganisms and other environmental agents that could cause allergic reactions or infections. The duration of the condition, severity and type of the conjunctivitis may vary. It may affect one eye only or both. It is easy to spread viral conjunctivitis through physical contact.

Conjunctivitis may also be caused by measles, colds, or respiratory infections. You will feel severe discomfort in your eyes, reddening of the whites, swelling of the eyelids, watery discharge, and irritation. Viral conjunctivitis might last up two weeks.

2. Astigmatism

Astigmatism can be one of most common eye conditions. Astigmatism can cause blurred vision because the cornea is unable to properly focus the image onto a retina.

A misaligned cornea can cause ineffectiveness when focusing light. The cornea looks more like a sphere. However, astigmatics may find their corneas to be elliptically shaped like a football.

Blurred vision and eye strain are the main symptoms of astigmatism. Eyestrain, headaches and eye pain are other common symptoms.

3. Glaucoma

Glaucoma is an eye condition that can cause complete blindness. Glaucoma is actually one of many leading causes of blindness. This could have been avoided. The optic nerve can be damaged if it is not treated.

We discussed the parts and functions of the eye in the previous chapter. In that chapter we also covered the aqueous humor. This is the watery substance which fills the eye. The ciliary tissues in the vicinity are responsible for continuously producing aqueoushumor and a system drainage canals removes it from the eye.

Glaucoma can develop when the aqueous fluid is not removed from the eyes quickly or if it is produced at a rapid rate, leading to pressure buildup. This pressure increase can alter the shape and degrade the optic nerve, leading to blind spots.

4. Macular degeneration

This can lead to the loss of vital retina parts called the macula. The macula, a region of the retina measuring three to five millimeters in size, is responsible central vision. Macular Degeneration results in irreversible loss and/or impairment of central vision. This means that you may not be able to see the centre of an object while still being able to see the perimeter.

Early signs of this condition may cause blurred, distorted and gray vision. Legal blindness is also a common condition for those over sixty. It affects a large number of seniors, with the most common being age-related maculopathy (ARMD).

ARMD is a common symptom of aging. Genes are also a factor. ARMD is more likely in people who have ARMD family members. The incidence of cases involving women is higher than that of males.

Central vision impairments are a sign of macular damage. You may notice, for instance, a blank spot when you read. Distortion of vision may also be experienced by the person (e.g. Straight lines that are bent. Stimuli could also appear smaller.

5. Retinitis pigmentosa

Retinitis Pigmentosa is another condition that eventually leads blindness. This disorder is caused mostly by the abnormalities in the visual nerves (mainly the rods) found within the retina.

The rods can be used for night vision as well as scotopic vision and peripheral sight. However, the cones can be used for sharp, central vision and color vision. The fovea is an area in which cones are usually clumped together. On the other hand, the rods are located around the fovea.

Retinitis pigmentosa is a condition that causes the rods to deteriorate. This makes it difficult for the patient to see in dim lighting and eventually leads to night vision loss. As the condition worsens, the rods become more affected. The rods also cause tunnel vision. As RP worsens, a person with it will lose a little of their central vision.

Retinitis pigmentosa can also be hereditary, just like macular damage. Unlike ARMD in which most cases involve older people, symptoms of RP may begin as early as adolescence. RP has no known treatment. RP can be treated by both medication and surgery. It is believed that vitamins can slow the development of RP.

6. Myopia

Myopia, also known as nearsightedness, refers to a condition in which the eye sees more clearly when stimuli are closer than those that are further away. Myopia can make far objects look blurred or fuzzy for myopic people. Reading a book is no problem for someone with myopia. However, looking at signage that is only a few metres away can be difficult.

Myopia is caused by the elongation and spherical shape of the eyeball. Normal eyes are spherical, but myopic ones have an oblong eyeball. In reality, most people are born with farsightedness. As we age, however, our hyperopia or farsightedness diminishes.

Myopia can be inherited from presbyopia. Myopia can develop in children as young a 5 year old.

7. Presbyopia

Presbyopia can be described as a condition where the eye becomes unable to see near objects. Presbyopia isn't a disease. It is normal and part of aging. Presbyopia will eventually develop over the years. By age 40, symptoms are common.

Presbyopia is mostly caused by the lens. The lens, located behind the iris or the pupil, is responsible for 20% eye's focusing ability. The lens' curvature, pulled and pushed by the ciliary muscle, is adjusted to bring objects in focus. As people age, the power of the ciliary muscle to pull and push the lens is diminished and the lens itself becomes less flexible and elastic. These changes in the lens and the ciliary muscles can cause the lens to not be adjusted for different distances. The effect would be that stimuli close to the person appear blurry.

Ever noticed your parents squinting at their phones as they read text messages? Presbyopia means that people over 50 would have difficulty reading text messages on their phones or in newspapers. Presbyopia may also be characterized by blurry or blurry vision and eyestrain from working close to the eyes.

8. Cataract

This is caused by cloudiness in your lens. It is usually transparent and clear. This can lead to vision difficulties and even blindness.

Understanding how cataracts form is easier if you know that the lens is made up of protein and water. As we age, our lens protein composition changes. These changes and alterations in water, enzymes, or other chemicals can lead to cataract formation.

The elderly are the most susceptible to developing cataracts, according to their age. Cataract can even be considered part and parcel of aging. If cataracts are linked to aging, it is more likely that they will occur in both of your eyes.

Poor central vision, blurry vision and frequent prescription changes are some of the symptoms of cataracts. There is also a milky white appearance in the pupil that can be caused by the development of the cataract.

9. Corneal abrasion

This condition is caused by direct injury to your eye. This could be caused by external elements, cosmetic items, such as contact lenses or makeup brushes, or even fingernail damage. Patients who have suffered from corneal erosion report feeling a foreign object in their eye, pain and tearing.

10. Corneal ulcer

Corneal inflammation is the cause of corneal ulcer. This inflammation is due to injury and infection.

Germs are the leading reason for corneal ulcer progression. However, germs will not normally enter a healthy cornea that has a functioning lid and adequate tears. Infections can occur when the eye's defense mechanisms are damaged.

The cornea can become inflamed or injured from many different situations. Contact lenses that are not properly used can cause eye injury. Malfunctioning tears ducts is another cause, as tears contain enzymes that protect the eye from infection.

Chapter 15: Good Vision With Proper Diet

Because your body can't function properly without food, it is important that you have enough food each day to sustain it. Contrary to popular belief however, you can't just eat anything. It is not enough that we eat whatever we want. To stay healthy, it is important to eat well. Your overall health can be directly affected by what you eat and how it's prepared. Your vision is the same. Your eyes are a vital part your body. Therefore, they are exposed to the effects that food has on them. When your mother told you to eat your carrots while you were young, you should have believed her. You shouldn't underestimate the importance of carrots, and other vegetables, in maintaining healthy eyesight.

Natural ways to improve your eyesight include eating a healthy and balanced diet. The best food can help preserve your vision. It can delay or prevent serious eye diseases, reduce the likelihood of developing them and even prevent some from happening.

There are many foods that have been found to have beneficial effects on eyesight. These benefits can be explained by vitamins, minerals and microelements in the foods. It is essential to learn about the different vitamins and minerals to determine which foods should be included in your daily meal plans.

Nutrients for Healthy Vision

Vitamins, organic chemical compounds, are required by the body for proper function. While only a small amount are necessary, they are essential in many of the major processes and systems in the body. A lack of vitamins can result in sickness or diseases. Since the body is not able to produce enough vitamins on its own, we must supplement them with foods that naturally contain them.

Minerals refer to solid chemical compounds that are created by geological processes. While soil and rocks can be rich in minerals it doesn't mean that you have to eat them to obtain them. Instead, we eat those animals and plants who have taken in minerals through the water they drank or food they ate.

Essential fatty oils are essential to healthy eyesight. Essential fatty acids such as omega 3 fatty acids and omega 6 are beneficial to the body. They aid in many bodily process. As vitamins cannot make enough of fatty acids, it is necessary to consume fatty foods. Particularly, the fatty acid I mentioned is important for your eye vision.

I will be discussing some of these vitamins, minerals, and essential fatty acids in the next section. This promotes healthier vision.

1. Vitamin C

Vitamin C is very important for normal eyesight. Vitamin C can be found in many fruits. It lowers the chances of developing cataracts as well as age-related macular disease (ARMD). Vitamin C is found in tomatoes, papaya and strawberries.

2. Vitamin E

Vitamin E is crucial for protecting eyes from damage caused by unstable molecules called free radicals. Vitamin E is considered a powerful antioxidant. It can be found in vegetable oil like corn oil, almond nuts, sunflower seeds, and safflower oils.

3. Vitamin A

Vitamin B1 is important for healthy vision development in children. It helps maintain normal function of your retina. Vitamin A is why carrots are highly recommended to children. It and other brightly colored fruits and vegetables contain the necessary vitamin. You can get Vitamin A by eating mangos squash, sweet potatoes and apricots.

4. Zinc

Zinc is recommended to naturally improve your eyesight. It is capable of transporting Vitamin A from the liver into the retinas of the eyes, to compensate for Vitamin A deficiency. Include zinc-rich foods, such as eggs, milks, shellfish, peanuts and beef, lamb, oysters and whole grains in your diet.

5. Lutein & zeaxanthin

Carotenoids, also known as natural coloring agents, include lutein and zeaxanthin. Carotenoids are natural coloring agents that aid plants in converting sunlight to nutrients. Zeaxanthin and lutein can be found in the eyes of people to help protect them from UV (ultraviolet) light. These nutrients decrease over time and require replenishment through deep yellow or green foods like broccoli, spinach, corn, and other vegetables.

6. Omega 3 Fatty Acids

All fats may not be bad. French fries made with fat Bad. Fat that aids in absorption of vitamins? Good. Fishes such as salmon, tuna, and trout are rich in Omega 3 fatty acid so make sure to include them in your diet.

These vitamins and minerals could help your eyes. The goal should be to find nutrients that can benefit your eyes every day. Research has shown, for example, that proper nutrition can reduce the risk of age-related macular disease or even slow down its progression. Doctors suggest that patients consume beta carotene or zinc as a precaution. Foods rich in antioxidants are also beneficial. Antioxidants can be described as carotene, betacarotene, or the mixture of carotenoids. These carotenoids are precursors for vitamins C, E, A and Z, selenium, zinc, and vitamin E. Foods rich in antioxidants include nuts, seeds and citrus fruits as well blueberries, cherries and yellow vegetables.

A healthy diet can also help prevent the development of other eye conditions.

Now that you know how important diet plays in maintaining healthy eyesight, it's time to change your lifestyle if you don't feel like you're making a difference for the good of your vision and your overall health.

For your Vision, Plan a Healthy Diet

A healthy diet is more than what you eat. You must also consider what you eat and how many.

Your diet needs to be balanced. It doesn't mean you have to eat only carrots, just because Vitamin A is important in improving your eye sight. Keep in mind that your diet is not only for your eyes, but also for your health. The ratio of food from different food groups can have an impact on your health. Therefore, it is important that you make sure you are consuming enough food from each food group.

A healthy diet that includes grain foods is good for you. These foods contain iron, B-vitamins, and dietary Fibers which support all systems of the body and aid in eye function. There are two kinds of grain foods, whole grains and processed grains. Whole-wheat flour, whole-wheat flour, brown rice, and oatmeal are all examples of whole grains. Refined grains include white bread, white rice and white flour. Whole grains are healthier than both types of grain foods. They have retained all their vitamins and minerals. Whole grains, unlike refined grains that cause rapid digestion and spikes in blood sugar levels, are slow to digest. This is good news for eyesight.

Vegetables are a fantastic source of nutrients. Make sure you eat them instead of throwing them out. Vegetables should always be included in your meal. Varieties of colors can help you choose the right vegetables for you. You can include carrots (kale), tomatoes, cucumbers, tomatoes, celery and celery in your daily diet.

Fruits are, like vegetables and other fruits, a great natural source for vitamins and minerals. You can benefit from it for your eyes and general well-being. Blueberries, kiwis, lemons, apples and avocados are some of the fruits that can help with healthy vision.

Dairy products like milk can provide your body with tons of nutrients. Low-fat natural milk products are better for your eyesight. Avoid sweetened milk products.

Also, protein should be included in your daily diet. You can find many nutrients that are beneficial for your eyes that only come from protein-rich foods. Fish is a great source of omega 3 fat acids. Good sources of lutein (and zeaxanthin) are eggs, while beef is good for zinc. You should eat lean cuts and avoid processed foods if you want to be healthy. You may be able to get sick from processed meat sources like sausages and ham.

Second, moderation is key. No matter how healthy your diet is, you will still be unable to enjoy the benefits of eating well-balanced food. No matter how varied or balanced your diet, if you are not getting enough nutrients for your body, it does not matter. It can be harmful for your health to eat too many of them.

Exercising too often can make you overweight. Overeating can lead to various health issues, such as diabetes and cardiovascular disease. This could also contribute to the progression of many eye disorders. Your body is more likely to contract infections and other diseases if you are underweight. Insufficient food intake is also a sign that your body is not receiving the proper nutrients for your eyes.

Here are some tips to help you eat in moderation.

1. Smaller portions are better

Reduce your portions to avoid overeating. Perhaps you can reduce your food intake by eating smaller portions at home. You should avoid ordering huge meals or main dishes when outside. It is also possible to share meals with others. However, fruits and veggies are something you can enjoy as much or as little as you wish.

2. Don't overeat

It is okay to occasionally overeat, but it will be more harmful to continue doing so regularly. Think about why you are overeating. Are you stressed? Are you tired? Only once you know the reason for your overeating, can you treat it.

3. You should not eat if your stomach is full.

Avoid eating outside of your regular mealtimes and when you are hungry, except if you are eating fruit or vegetables. What about snacking while you're watching TV and lazing around? Nope. This is a bad idea. Do not eat at the same time.

Avoid certain foods

To be able to see clearly, you need to know which foods are good for your eyes. Your eyes will suffer if you eat foods that are not good for your health. These are the foods you should avoid for your health.

1. Junk foods

This includes chips, candy, and any other processed food. Junk food generally has a very negative impact on the human body. Junk food contains a lot of sugar, salt, fats and can lead to many health problems including those related to the eyes.

2. Deep-fried food

It is true that you included all the recommended protein foods in a healthy diet, but you deep-fried the food. Your food is going to end up being unhealthy. It's not just the type of food that matters, but also how you prepare it for consumption. The food structure is affected by deep frying. You also lose the nutritional value of your food by using this method of cooking. Eating too many deep-fried foods can increase the number of free radicals that can cause eye damage and accelerate aging. Sweet potatoes, which are rich in nutrients, are good for healthy eyesight. But, by deep-frying them, you ruin their vitamin content and add harmful fats to the oil.

3. Foods high in sugar

Your eyes are at risk if your blood sugar levels spike. This is why eye conditions like diabetes are often linked with diabetes. Consuming high levels of sugar should be avoided.

Chapter 16: Vision And Exercise

Vision relaxation techniques are one of the most effective ways to naturally improve your eyesight. Do not be worried. Do not worry about what you read. Visual exercises and relaxation techniques can be easily done. They are designed to help with the most common conditions of the eyes and can be done frequently to improve your vision.

Some people might doubt the effectiveness of these exercises. It might seem easy to determine which technique is best for your eyes. There are visual exercises that can't be supported by scientific evidence. However, there have been many examples of real-life results that show the benefits they have.

Also, it is not absurd to believe that visual exercises are highly effective. With the introduction of yoga, relaxation is a proven method for improving health and wellbeing. There is no conclusive scientific evidence to show yoga exercises has a positive effect on your health. However, there are many other benefits.

Another benefit of vision exercises is their accessibility and affordability. They are much more affordable than corrective glasses or surgeries, and they don't require any expense.

Eye relaxation techniques

Our eyes are subject to a lot of stress. Most of us work for long hours every week. Please don't tell my that you aren't using your eyes while working. For those who are working close-up or exposed to gadgets, the strain on their eyes is immense. We only get to rest our eyes when we sleep. There are days when you only get to rest for two to three hour a night.

It is essential to rest in order to maintain the body's normal function. How much rest we get can have a significant impact on our physical health, psychological well-being, and emotional well being. This is true also for our eyes.

Eye relaxation can have many benefits. For example, taking a few moments to rest your eyes every now and again not only gives your eyes a break but also allows your mind and body to recharge. To feel refreshed, it is worth closing your eyes and taking in a deep breathe.

Eye relaxation also benefits other systems.

You can easily relax your eyes with the many eye relaxation techniques that are available.

1. Palming eye technique

You can use the palming eye technique by sitting down on a stool and making yourself comfortable. Once you are comfortable, move your hands to the sides and rub them together. You will then close your eyes. Next, cover your eyes with your hands. Continue to take deep breaths at regular intervals after you've completed the previous step. Do this for approximately five minutes.

2. Acupuncture Technique

This eye relaxation technique can be used by people who work closely with computers, or do close-up work. Before you begin this massage technique, be sure to make sure your fingernails don't become too sharp. You will need to sit down comfortably in your chair. Begin by laying down on your back. You can do this by using circular motions. Next, move onwards to the areas below your pupils. You can then move to the last massage points at your temples. Continue the same circular motions. The whole massage should last at least five minutes.

3. Green Therapy

This is probably the easiest technique to use. Simply spend some time looking at something green in the distance. It is so refreshing to see green. Stop working for a while and take a look outside at the tree, or at a nearby houseplant.

Vision exercises

The primary purpose of vision exercises is to reduce the symptoms of common eye disorders, such as nearsightedness or farsightedness.

The first thing to understand about vision exercises is their effectiveness. The type of disorder and the individual's lifestyle will have an impact on how quickly and how far the eyesight will improve.

One of the biggest benefits of vision exercises is the ability to reduce vision stress. Vision stress is one contributing factor to the development or eye problems. A reduction in vision stress can lead to better vision. Vision exercises are a great way to do this.

I will be introducing some vision exercises that will help you naturally improve your eyesight. You should not force yourself into doing them. You can always stop if any of these exercises causes your eyes to hurt or leads to mental fatigue. For the duration of these exercises, please put aside your eyeglasses.

1. Infinity Figure Vision Exercise

This eye exercise can help you strengthen your eyes muscles and make them flexible. All you have to do is locate a wall. Three steps from your wall, place your chair. This distance should be about ten feet. Next, imagine a huge infinity sign, or figure 8, that is placed horizontally on the wall infront. After you have finished that, start to trace the outline with your eyes the infinity symbol. You have the option to choose where you start, as long as it is slow and you don't move your head. You can stop and rest your eyes for a few moments after you've completed the infinity sign in one direction. Then, go back and do it the other way. Repeat the exercise five times.

It is possible for your eyes to feel tired before you are able to trace the infinity symbols five times. Don't panic. Keep at it. Repetition is a great way to increase your repetitions.

2. Candle Vision Exercise

This visual exercise targets those who suffer from hyperopia or farsightedness. You will need to light a candle and place it on a table. You will then need to place your feet on the table so that the flame of the candle is not too close to your eyes. The candlelight should be approximately four feet away from you. Also, your spine and neck should remain straight as you sit down. After you have completed all preparations, move on to the next step. Focus your eyes on the candlelight one minute and stare at it without blinking. Do not close your eyes, or move away from candlelight. You should not panic if your eyes water. After the one-minute, close your eyes. Now imagine the candlelight in your head. Imagine the flame being between your eyebrows. You can hold on to this image for as long and as you like. Once you are done, you can again open your eyes and gaze at the candlelight. This process should be repeated at least five times.

3. Two Dots Exercise

This type of exercise can be very beneficial for strengthening the muscles in your eyes. This exercise is recommended for people who work near computers or have close-up jobs. Like the infinity exercises, locate a wall and stand ten feet from it. Imagine two dots that are roughly one and half meters apart on the wall. Take a deep breathe. If distance is difficult to judge, you can create these dots using colored circles. Then pin the medium-sized circles to the wall. Continue to stare at one of the dots for several seconds, then shift your focus to the other.

You can then look at the second dot again for a few seconds, before slowly moving your attention back to the original dot. For approximately three minutes, you can complete this exercise before closing your eyes.

4. Blinking exercise

Blinking is an unconsciously performed reflex that involves rapid eyelid opening and closing. This seemingly insignificant action can have a positive impact on our eye health. Every time we blink, tears are produced to moisturize the eye and remove any irritants.

Normally, a healthy person blinks twelve to fifteen times per hour. But we blink less when we're focused on something. Blinking can be reduced to 3 to 5 times per minute for those who focus on a task that requires concentration such as reading, working on a laptop, watching TV, and so forth. This is not recommended, as it can lead to dry eyes and cause strain on the eyes.

It is also important to practice blinking to maintain your eye's health. This can be done by taking off any eyewear. Close your eyes for a few seconds, then relax them. Now, close your eyes and blink 15 times fast. You should not add any tension to your eyes or face. Let your eyes blink lightly, and you will see that your eyelids resemble the wings of butterflies. Close your eyes, and blink for 15 times. Then relax. Repeat the entire procedure twice.

5. Exercise for up-and-down eye movement

This exercise is intended to alleviate eyestrain. There are many reasons that eyestrain may occur. When you work for a while on your computer, reading, or other tasks that require your eyes to be focused for an extended period of time, you may feel headaches, blurred sight, and trouble focusing. These happen because your eyes are overworked. This exercise will help to relieve eye strain and can also be used as a preventive measure. It is important to first get comfortable on the chair you choose. You need to ensure your neck, spine, and face remain relaxed. Be sure to keep your back straight. After taking a deep inhale, you can face forward and continue looking straight ahead. Next, try to raise your eyes as high as you can. Try to imagine something between your eyebrows. Then, open your eyes and move them upwards. After you have completed the previous step move your eyes down, as far downward as you can, and imagine that this time you are trying to reach your mouth. Now, look straight ahead to return your eyes to their normal position.

Keep your breathing steady as you go through the steps. Your muscles should be as relaxed as possible, and you should maintain a straight neck.

Chapter 17: Vision And Lifestyle Improvements

Recent trends have led to people being more aware of their own health. Millions have joined yoga classes to lose weight and relax since the advent of yoga. Too focused on external appearances can lead to neglect of internal processes and other body parts. One of the most neglected parts of our bodies is the eyes. The visual process, for instance, is something we often forget about. We assume we will still be able see until our death and that any changes to our vision will occur in the future. Visual disorders aren't limited to the elderly, as we have seen. Our actions can lead to visual problems early in life. This is because health issues are not just the result of genetic predispositions. But lifestyle can also play a role. Lifestyle factors have a significant impact on our vision quality. This chapter will focus on lifestyle changes that you can make, other than changing your diet, to improve your eyesight naturally and make it better.

Be active

Eyesight can be affected by a lack or activity. Inactive people have a greater chance of developing age-related retinal degeneration. Lack of movement can have the biggest impact on the body.

For eyesight improvement and general wellbeing, it is recommended to do at least three exercises per week.

Good hygiene is important.

Stop smoking.

Smoking increases your chance of developing damage to the optic neuron, cataracts and macular disease. Smokers must stop smoking as soon possible.

Regulate alcohol intake.

Smoking and alcohol consumption have been linked to several eye conditions. You need to be careful about how much alcohol you consume.

You can rest your eyes.

Eyes can also experience fatigue, just as any other part of the body. If you've ever been on your computer for too long, you may notice that you have headaches and eye pain. This happens because if your eyes strain too much, stress can manifest itself in the form of headaches and eye pain.

Below I'll be sharing some tips and tricks to help you see better.

1. Set text size.

Because people are now so attached to their computers it is more likely they spend a lot of time staring at them than looking at other things. Adjust your settings to make text larger when you look at something in your computer.

2. Adjust brightness.

You can take note of the lighting in your area and decide how bright it looks. When you are working in a room, take a look at the lighting and determine if it is adequate or too bright. How bright is the lamp? Are you forced to look at the letters with your eyes closed to be able see them? To help your eyes, you should take the appropriate steps to make your environment brighter or more pleasant.

It would be a great idea to turn the brightness down if you are using the TV or computer.

3. Make sure to blink.

Laptop users may notice a tendency to blink less when using other electronic gadgets. This will lead to dryness at the eye surface. The result is a burning, irritating sensation. When using your gadgets, remember to keep the normal blink rate of twelve to fifteen times per hour.

4. The 20-20-20 rule is a good idea.

The "20-20-20" trick is an eye exercise which can help your eyes rest for some time. Take a 20 minute break if you have to be looking at a screen or paper for a long time. For at least 20 seconds, fix your eyes on a point about 20 feet away. This will help your eyes as well as your entire body.

Wear protective eyewear.

Some people find wearing protective eyewear annoying. It all depends on the situation. You need to learn how to protect your eyes to avoid corneal erosion and other serious conditions.

Safety glasses or protective goggles are essential if your work involves exposure to hazardous materials. If you are working on construction sites, don't compromise your safety for the sake or aesthetics.

Sports enthusiasts should wear helmets if their sport requires them.

Avoid the use of contact lenses.

Contact lenses offer many benefits to their wearers. They can cause eye infection if not properly used. Corneal abrasion can be caused by improperly wearing contact lenses. You should not wear contact lenses unless your eye physician has recommended it. This can increase the chance of developing dry eye or other eye conditions that can affect vision.

Wear correct eye prescription.

Do not remove your current eyeglasses in the hope that your vision will improve. If your eye doctor suggests any course of action (e.g. You should wear your eyeglasses. It is essential that you wear the correct prescription for your eyes. There are many people out there who didn't bother to see their eye doctor and bought eyeglasses with the prescription that best suits their eyes. This can cause serious problems, since wearing eyeglasses with too high or too small prescriptions will not only affect your eyesight but could even make things worse.

You should also address other medical issues.

Healthy eyesight can also be achieved by taking care your other health issues. It is possible to prevent eye conditions from developing if you address other health concerns. Astigmatism has been linked to diabetes. Eyes may become blurred if there are changes in the shape or blood sugar levels. While this process can be slow, it is better to control your sugar intake to avoid developing astigmatism.

Visit your eye doctor regularly.

Your eye doctor should see you and perform tests to identify if there are any signs or symptoms that could indicate a possible eye disorder. Preventive measures can be taken to stop the disorder from progressing fully. This is a wise move.

Always be safe with your eyes.

Good hygiene is important.

Proper hygiene is crucial to keep your eyes healthy. When you touch your eyelids, make sure you wash your hands often with antiseptic soap. You should avoid any allergens, as they could trigger a reaction that could lead to pinkeye or other complications.

At the end of each day, remove any makeup, particularly eye makeup. Avoid touching your eyes if possible. In cases where you have itchy eyelids, don't touch them.

Apply a warm compress to your eyes every now and again. Warm compresses can be used to clean the eye area and improve the condition. A warm compress applied several times daily is an effective way to reduce the discomfort of viral conjunctivitis.

Structures of your eyes

The protective, opaque and fibrous outer layer that covers the eye (the sclera) acts as a barrier.

The pupil is a hole in the centre iris that allows light to enter. It allows light in the eye. The pupil appears darkened because light rays entering its pupil are absorbed in the tissues of the eye. You can have them absorbed after they are scattered throughout the eye.

The Iris (a thin, circular component in the pupil) is located within the eye's lens. It regulates the pupil's diameter and shape. The term colour of iris refers to the color of your eyes.

The Cornea (transparent area in front of the eye) protects all three areas: the anterior chamber and iris. The cornea acts in conjunction with the anterior and lens to refract light. This mechanism accounts roughly for around two-thirds to the total optical power in the eye.

The crystalline lenses is a clear structure having a biconvex design. Together with the cornea it aids in light refraction, allowing light to be focused onto the retina. The lens changes the focal distance of your eye by altering its shape. This is so that it can focus on objects at different distances.

The retina, which is a thin layer on the retina that detects light and lines the cornea of the eye, is a light-sensitive tissue. It collects light through the cornea, crystalline lens and other parts of the eye. This is followed by the generation images by evoking nerve impulses. These impulses travel through the optic nerve to the visual part of the brain.

The macula (or fovea) are important parts in the vision. Both are small areas on the retina that are covered with rods and conicals.

The Most Common Causes of Vision loss

You should get a thorough examination by your eye doctor. Your medical history and prescriptions are all important to an optometrist. To determine if natural therapy is the right path to your vision health, please consider the following reasons for vision impairment:

Bacterial contamination

Medications

Scars on the cornea

Tumors of eye

Retinitis

Diabetes-related Retinopathy

Glaucoma

Macular degeneration with age

Cataracts

Trauma

An insufficient intake of vitamin A

Viral infection of the eyes

Poisoning or Toxins

Low vision increases with age and may be more frequent. These conditions can have an impact on brain visual processing areas. It is not blindness. Eyeglasses cannot correct it.

Although it does not require a large investment to promote eye health, it does make sense to research what works and what doesn't. Avoiding cigarette smoking, wearing sunglasses when outdoors, and eating healthy meals that are nutrient-dense are simple ways to prevent vision damage. These are all factors that can impact our eyesight.

Vitamins and minerals are essential for good health.

Macular degeneration can be prevented by taking antioxidants such as vitamin A, C, E and zinc. It's a condition where the macula -- which is the part of the eye that regulates central sight -- becomes blurred, making it hard to see clearly.

There are many colourful vegetables and fruits that provide these essential nutrients, including the following:

Combining red peppers and carrots is a wonderful combination.

broccoli florets, spinach leaves, strawberries

Supplemental eye health can be improved by eating sweet potatoes and citrus, as well as omega-3 fatty foods like flaxseed and salmon.

Don't forget the carotene content.

You will also need to take in a few extra nutrients to improve your eyesight. There are two carotenoids lutein & zeaxanthin that are high in retinal pigment. They can also be found among other foods such as eggs, broccoli, zucchini and leafy green veggies.

Supplements with lutein and/or zeaxanthin also are available. They work by increasing the pigment density in macula and absorption of ultraviolet and blue lights in that part.

Maintain your physical fitness at an elite level.

Yes, maintaining a healthy weight and exercising regularly may be good for your eyes. Type 2 Diabetes, more common in obese than in healthy people may lead to damage of the tiny blood vessels in your eyes.

Diabetic retinalopathy is the medical name used to describe this condition. High levels of sugar in your bloodstream can damage the weak arterial walls. Diabetic retinopathy, which is caused by the fluid and blood flowing into the retina (the light-sensitive back part of the eye), can cause vision problems.

You can reduce your chance of developing type 2, diabetes, and other complications by regularly having your blood sugar levels checked.

Maintain good health for chronic diseases

Vision problems may not be caused solely by diabetes. Not all medical conditions that can affect your eyesight such as multiple sclerosis or high blood pressure are fully understood. These conditions may be related to chronic inflammation which can have negative effects on your health from head-to-toe.

It is possible for an optic nerve to become inflamed, which can cause pain or complete vision loss. Multiple sclerosis, although it is not preventable, can be controlled with the right practices and medications.

For high blood pressure treatment, it is important to eat a healthy diet and exercise regularly.

10 Amazing Herbs for Eyecare

Many people believe that nature has the power to cure any condition or illness. However, there are some plants that can assist you with your vision issues. For thousands of years herbs have been used as a treatment for various ailments. Here are some herbs that could help to improve or strengthen your eyesight.

Bentonite-based poultices

Bentonite is a great natural treatment for eye strain. It works by removing any pollutants from the eye.

Fennel

You can use it to make tea or to clean your eyes. Fennel's antioxidant vitamins A & C help prevent macular deterioration.

Additionally, the minerals found in fennel can help prevent cataracts deterioration.

Passionflower

This plant extract is great for relieving eye strain. It also acts as a nerve relaxing agent. It has been found to relax blood vessels in eyes. Passionflower is also beneficial for treating eye conditions such as heart disease, burns, ADHD and asthma. It is also used for treating earache and boils.

Jaborandi

Glaucoma sufferers will appreciate the benefits of this plant. It can be very helpful in the early stages. Apply the oil of Jaborandi directly to the affected eye. This should bring relief.

Bilberry

This plant is great for improving your night vision. A supplement made from this plant could help you see better at night if you have trouble driving.

It can also be used for menstruation cramps.

Asphalt

South African Bushmen have been using this plant for thousands years to improve their vision and immune system. It is rich with calcium, iron zinc, antioxidants, magnesium and zinc.

Grapeseed extract

It's an immune-boosting and vision-enhancing plant. It improves the retina.

One research suggests that Grape Seed Extract may help in the treatment and prevention or Alzheimer's Disease.

Gingko Biloba (Gingko Biloba)

This is a traditional treatment to increase circulation in the area behind one's eye. It improves blood flow throughout the eye by increasing its circulation.

Gingko has also been shown to be helpful in memory-related diseases such as Alzheimer's and dementia. It is also used for multiple sclerosis, tinnitus, and other conditions.

Bilwa

It is used for conjunctivitis, sty, and other eye conditions. This plant is rich source of protein, pectin as well minerals such iron, phosphorus calcium, magnesium and other minerals.

It is often used in cold beverages. This extract is combined with water and sugar to make a healthy, delicious beverage that benefits your vision.

The Golden Seal

It has been shown to be beneficial in reducing inflammation and eye discomfort. To treat eye infections, you can make an eyewash from it.

Berberine accounts for the effectiveness the Golden Seal. It is a chemical which is capable of killing fungi and germs. It also has characteristics that can maintain a normal pulse, and lower blood pressure.

Ayurvedic Eye Improvement Remedies

Ayurveda could be the most basic and natural way to improve your vision. Here are the ways Ayurveda might help you enhance your sight.

Poor vision is now a common issue in our modern world. It can be either nearsightedness, or farsightedness. People are using glasses and contact lenses to correct their vision problems. Who would want to wear glasses? However, most of these people don't wear glasses. They should, however. We don't love the idea of using eye drops or medications to improve our vision. You have no other options for improving your vision. There is an alternative that can help. Ayurveda is for you! Ayurveda calls poor eyesight Drishti dosha. It can be caused by neurological issues, intestinal issues, congestion, or neurological debility.

Almond

Almonds' natural Omega-3 fatty acids and vitamin E as well as antioxidants can naturally improve your vision. They improve memory and focus. Almonds can be eaten as-is or made into a paste with soaked almonds. You can also drink the paste with a glass o milk. For a few months or until your health improves, you can continue doing this daily.

Asparagus wild

It is used in Ayurveda. Wild asparagus is a great plant for improving vision. This plant can help increase vision and extend life expectancy. You can mix a spoonful with honey of wild asparagus, and then drink it daily with a cup warm cow's milk. For several months, you can do this again.

The Indian gooseberry herb is called amla.

Amla is a well-known Ayurvedic medicine that enhances vision. Indian gooseberry is often called amla. It's one of the richest source of vitamin C. This fruit is rich with antioxidants, and other powerful ingredients that may improve your vision. Vitamin C is found in amla, which improves the function retinal cells. This can be done by adding a few spoonfuls to half a glass of amla water. The juice should be taken twice daily, once in the morning and once in the evening. You can also make the juice with honey, and have it as a snack.

Wear protective eyewear

Protect your eyes whenever you are working in your garden, playing racquetball, or conducting a scientific experiment at school.

Wearing tough protective eyewear is important when chemicals, sharp blades, and other materials can enter your eyes.

Polycarbonate is used for the production of large quantities of protective eyewear because it is around 10 times more strong than other forms.

This category includes sunglasses.

Sunglasses go beyond fashion and style. They protect your eyes from damaging UV rays. To improve your eyesight, sunglasses are a must. It is also the most affordable. It is excellent for blocking UVA/UVB radiation.

You may find that sunglasses are beneficial for protecting your eyes from vision damage. Pterygium is a condition where tissue grows over the white of the eyeball. Cataracts and Pterygium are other examples. Pterygiums can cause astigmatism. This is characterized with fuzzy vision.

It may be beneficial to protect your eyes from sunburn by wearing a hat with wide brim.

Use the 20-20-20 Rule as often as you can.

Your eyes work very hard all the time and need to be given a break once in a while. Stress levels rise when you spend too much time on a computer. It is important to follow the 20-20-20 Rule in order to reduce tension.

It is a good idea to take a 20-second break every 20 mins and look at everything 20 feet away for 20 secs.

You can live longer if you quit smoking.

You already know that smoking can be bad for your lungs and heart. It is important to include your eyes in this. Your risk of developing cataracts, age-related macular disease and other eye problems is greatly increased by smoking cigarettes.

If you've had years of nicotine-induced damage to your eyes or lungs, heart, liver, and other bodily functions, you may notice an improvement within the first few days after quitting. The more time you can avoid smoking, the better your blood vessels will be and the less inflammation you'll experience in your eyes as well as throughout your body.

Learn more about your family's history with eye disease and how they were treated.

You may be able to prevent certain eye conditions by knowing the family history of your grandparents.

Here are some examples:

Glaucoma is a sign of age-related macular and retinal disease. Optic atrophy can also be caused by age-related macular and retinal degeneration.

You may be able to take preventive steps by learning more about your family's history.

You should always keep your eyeglasses and hands as clean, as well as your eyes, as clean as you can.

Germs, infections, and other harmful substances can cause severe damage to your eyes. Sometimes, even small objects can cause vision problems. This can be avoided by always washing your hands before you touch your contact lenses.

Follow the instructions of your manufacturer for cleaning your hands and disinfecting contact lenses.

Also, it is important to replace your contacts lenses regularly as directed by the manufacturer and your physician. You might have bacterial infections from microorganisms in the lenses.

Your overall health and prevention of sickness are your responsibility.

It is important to keep in mind that eye diseases such as diabetes and high blood pressure may have an adverse effect on your eyesight over time. Certain diseases, such as optic nerve inflammation, can lead to vision loss and visual problems.

Understanding how to address these issues is key to avoiding further complications.

Some foods may help improve your vision

We all hope to have survived allergy season with our mental, physical and even our vision intact. Long roads to recovery have been traveled. Along with piles and bottles of nasal spray and vials filled with lubricating droplets to relieve dry eye discomfort, there has been much to be done. As it is tradition, allergies season is when eye appointments are most in demand.

Asheville locals know that local honey is one of their most effective allergy remedies. Although it is common knowledge that local honey can give your body the medicines it needs to fight and alleviate allergy symptoms, it isn't well-known. We're not surprised that we're open to local knowledge when it comes allergies. However we are less interested in using this expertise when it's about how to prevent dry eye, macular degeneration and even cataracts.

Most of us don't pay enough attention to our eyesight, and we forget about it until something goes wrong. We live in an age of "information overload", which has made life very stressful. The warning lights may not start flashing or beeping until we are aware that something is wrong. Eye problems can include blurred vision or headaches. However, a simple step can help reduce the severity of most eye problems.

Be mindful of what you are eating.

A simple, but effective way to protect your sight is to be mindful of what you are eating and to check what you are eating. We may not always be able to see the connection between our vision, what we eat for lunch, dinner, and breakfast. But we can. When we eat well, we are able to take better care of our vision and prevent the need for a visit to the eye doctor.

We wanted to make it easier for you by creating a list of foods high in antioxidants, which have powerful health-improving abilities. So, when you next go out to eat, or to the grocery store for your weekly meal plan, you will have a better idea about what you should add to your grocery shopping list.

Cold-water fish omega-3 fat acids (such as those found on fish, salmon and sardines) may help protect dry eyes and prevent macular degeneration. If you do eat fish, supplementing your omega-3 intake may be possible with fish oil or vegetarian supplements like flaxseed or black currant oil.

Vegetables with leafy greens

As two of the most important plant pigments, lutein (from spinach) and zeaxanthin (from kale), collard greens and kale have been shown to reduce macular degeneration as well as cataracts in certain people. This powerful antioxidant combination is also found in vegetables like broccoli, peas, avocados, and others.

Lutein, vitamin A, and vitamin B are just a few of the vitamins and mineral found in eggs. These vitamins and nutrients help maintain and improve eye function and health.

Grain is a cereal that can be grown in a field (Whole).

A higher intake of foods with low glycemic-index food (GI), may lower the likelihood of developing AMD. Replace processed carbohydrates with whole grains such as brown rice, whole oatmeal, whole oats, whole-wheat bread, pasta, and whole-wheat pieces. Whole grains contain vitamins E, zinc, as well as niacin. All of these are beneficial for the eyes in different ways.

Citrus and berries are two of the most nutritious fruits.

The high vitamin C content of citrus fruits, grapefruits, lemons and berries could help reduce the risk of macular degeneration.

You can also mention some foods high in vitamin E (omega-3 fatty acids) such as almonds, walnuts, and pistachios. These are all good for your eye health.

The high levels of bioflavonoids in lentils, kidney beans, black-eyed legumes and zinc in black-eyed and kidney beans may protect the retina. This could help lower the risk of developing eye diseases such as macular and cataracts.

Omega-3 fatty oils can be found within a wide range of foods, including fish oil (flaxseed oil) and black currant seed oil.

These omega-3 supplements have some positive effects on eyes health. They can prevent or treat dry eye syndromes and reduce the risk of developing macular degeneration.

Sunflower seeds are an example of a seed.

Sunflower seeds, rich in vitamin E as well as zinc, can help you maintain healthy eyes.

Beef

Consuming lean beef in moderation can be good for your eye health. Zinc in beef may aid in the absorption vitamin B and could help reduce the severity of age-related macular damage in the elderly.

More information on eye exercises: How to do them, their effectiveness, and what they do.

People have advocated eye exercises for hundreds of years as a natural remedy for a range of visual disorders, including weak eyesight. There is very little scientific evidence to support the claims that eye exercises may improve your vision. The benefits of exercises can be used to relieve eyestrain, improve your eyesight, and even help you see better.

Eye exercises may not be beneficial for people with chronic conditions like hyperopia (farsightedness), nearsightedness, or astigmatism. Most people who have common eye conditions like age-related macular damage, cataracts and glaucoma will find that eye exercises are not of any benefit.

While eye exercises may not improve your sight, they can make your eyes feel more relaxed. This is especially important for those who have eyes that get irritated from work.

Digital eye strain, also known computer vision syndrome, affects people who spend their days in front of computers. This illness can cause the following symptoms:

Eye strain, dry eyes, and reduced vision are all common causes of headaches.

A few simple exercises can help to relieve the symptoms of digital eyestrain.

How to get eyes to do their job

Depending on your specific needs, you might experiment with various eye exercises.

It is necessary for attention to be altered.

It is important to keep your attention focused due to the nature of this exercise. It is recommended to sit while working.

Keep a gap of at least a few inches between the tip of your finger and the eyeball when looking at anything.

Keep your attention on the finger holding you.

It's important to pay attention and not let your finger touch your face.

Take a few slow steps back and focus your gaze towards the horizon.

Continue to slowly shift your focus back to the extended finger. Then, return it to your eye.

Focus your attention away from the moment and instead, focus on something far away.

Repeat the process three more times until you are satisfied.

It is important to keep your eyes open for distant and immediate effects

The objective is to improve concentration. The task should be completed in the same sitting position as the previous.

For 15 seconds, maintain a distance between your thumbs and your face of about 10 inches.

For 15 seconds, focus on the object and determine its approximate location.

Your focus should be on your index finger.

Repetition the process five more times is a reasonable rule of thumb.

eighteenth illustration

Ideally, the exercise should be performed while you are sitting down.

Keep your eyes fixed about ten feet in front on a certain spot on the floor.

In your imagination, draw an eight-pointed figure with only your eyes.

For 30 seconds, keep going in the same direction.

How does vision therapy work? And how can you benefit from it?

Patients can seek the services of specialist doctors who specialize in vision therapy. In order to get the best results, eye exercises are sometimes used in vision therapy.

Some reports indicate that the goal of vision therapy may be to increase muscle strength in the eyes in particular circumstances. The researchers believe that it can also be used to retrain inappropriate visual behavior, as well as resolve eye-tracking irregularities. Vision therapy can be used in a number of conditions that are often seen in children. However, it can also be used in some cases to treat adult disorders. These are some examples of conditions:

Insufficiency in the viewpoint of convergence (CI).

Strabismus, also known as "stumbling block", is a condition that causes one's eye to cross (crosseye or walleye).

Amblyopia can be described as a condition in the eye that prevents a person from seeing (lazy-eye).

www.ingramcontent.com/pod-product-compliance
Lightning Source LLC
Chambersburg PA
CBHW060329030426
42336CB00011B/1266

* 9 7 8 1 7 7 4 8 5 9 7 1 1 *